MEMORY NOTEBOOK OF NURSING
Volume 2, 4th Edition

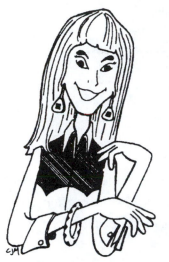

JoAnn Zerwekh, EdD, MSN, RN
President/CEO
Nursing Education Consultants
Chandler, AZ

Nursing Faculty
University of Phoenix
Phoenix, AZ

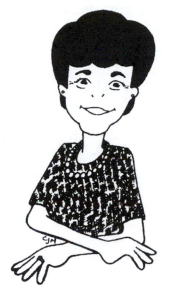

Jo Carol Claborn, MS, RN
Nurse Educator
Seymour, TX

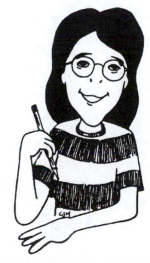

CJ Miller, RN, BSN
Nurse Illustrator
Iowa City, IA

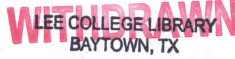

Artist: C.J. Miller, RN, BSN
Iowa City, Iowa

Production Manager: Mike Cull
Gingerbread Press, Waxahachie, Texas
Desktop Publishing: Lindy Nobles, Prosper, Texas

◆

◆

Printed in the United States of America

Nursing Education Consultants
P O Box 12200
Chandler, AZ 85248
800-933-7277
www.NursingEd.com

ISBN 1-892155-17-6   II ISBN   978-1-892155-17-7
LOC #: 2007939690

◆

Any procedure or practice described in this book should be applied by the health-care practitioner under appropriate supervision in accordance with professional standards of care used with regard to the unique circumstances that apply in each practice situation. Care has been taken to confirm the accuracy of information presented and to describe generally accepted practices. However, the authors, editors, and publisher cannot accept any responsibility for errors or omissions or for consequences from application of the information in this book and make no warranty, express or implied, with respect to the contents of this book.

This book is written to be used as a study aid and review book for nursing. It is not intended for use as a primary resource for procedures, treatments, medications or to serve as a complete textbook for nursing care.

Copies of this book may be obtained directly from Nursing Education Consultants.

Last Digit Is the Print Number: 6 5 4 3 2

CONTRIBUTORS

Joanna Barnes, MSN, RN
ADN Program Director
Grayson County College
Denison, TX

Deanne A. Blach, MSN, RN
Nurse Educator
President, DB Productions
Green Forest, AR

Tim Bristol, PhD, RN, CNE
NurseTim, Inc.
Executive Director
Waconia, MN

Sharon Decker, PhD, RN, ACNS-BC, ANEF
Professor and Director of Clinical Simulations
Covenant Health System Endowed Chair in Simulation
and Nursing Education
Texas Tech University Health Science Center
Lubbock, TX

Barbara Devitt, MSN, RN
Nursing Faculty
Louise Herrington School of Nursing
Baylor University
Dallas, TX

Shirley Greenway
Associate Degree Nursing Professor
Grayson County College
Denison, TX

Kisandra Harris, RN
Edmund, OK

Lt. Col. (Ret.) Michael W. Hutton, MSN, RN
Nursing Faculty
Blinn College
Bryan, TX

Alice Pappas, PhD, RN
Nurse Consultant
Norton, MA

Catherine Rosser, EdD, RN, CAN-BC,
Undergraduate Program Director
Louise Herrington School of Nursing
Baylor University
Dallas, TX

Elizabeth Kurczyn Valle, RN, BSN
Laredo Community College
Laredo, TX

Virginia "Ginny" Wangerin, RN, MSN, PhDc
Nurse Consultant, Educator
Administrator Emeritus, Des Moines Area
Community College

Mary Ann Yantis, BS, MS, PhD, RN
Faculty
Nursing Education Consultants, Inc.
Chandler, AZ

ACKNOWLEDGMENTS

From the authors: We want to express our appreciation to the students and faculty who have responded so positively to the Memory Notebook of Nursing, Vol 2. Through your support and contributions, this fourth edition was possible.

We wish to thank Robert Claborn and John Masog (our husbands) for their tolerance and sense of humor as we continued to work on revisions of another book! Also, we want to thank our 'adult children' Ashley Garneau and Tyler Zerwekh, Jaelyn Conway, Mike Brown, and Kim Aultman for their unconditional support and inspiration as we continue our journey in publishing.

From the illustrator: My work is dedicated to Nathan and Kim, the two best kids in the world and to my grandson Cohen. Without your love and support, I couldn't do what I do.

Our sincere appreciation to:

Lindy Nobles, our graphics production manager, whose exceptional technological skills contributed to the major revision of this project;

Elaine Nokes who has an amazing ability to organize our office and keep us on track with all that we do;

Dave Meier from the Center for Accelerated Learning at Lake Geneva, WI for introducing us to these ideas to help students learn.

PREFACE

Memory Notebook of Nursing, Volume 2, 4th edition is a new and different collection of memory tools, mnemonics, and visual images from *Memory Notebook of Nursing Vol. 1, 4th edition*. Your interest and enthusiasm with the third edition of the *Memory Notebook of Nursing* has encouraged us to produce a fourth edition. Nursing Education Consultants has taken your suggestions and ideas utilizing principles of accelerated learning along with the talents of an artist (who is also a nurse), C.J. Miller and incorporated them into this new edition. We have maintained this appealing and humorous approach to remembering important information. Many of these memory aids have been around since people first drew on the walls of caves and hence their origins are unknown. ☺

To assist you in the utilization of this book, here is a little information about accelerated learning and how you can enhance your learning by utilizing both the left (analytical, linear, logical, rote memory) side of your brain and the right (visual, images, musical, imaginative) side of your brain. Several techniques are used to encourage the whole-brain to think and learn concepts. These techniques are memory tools and mnemonics. Memory tools are aids to assist you to draw associations from other ideas with the use of visual images to help cement the learning. Mnemonics are most often words, phrases, or sentences that help you remember information. Throughout this book, you will find ideas that we have found useful in teaching students how to remember information. As you read over each illustration, get involved with the process and write down your own ideas on the drawings. Think about this, color activates the brain and music increases right brain activity. As you are coloring or writing, turn on some music, don't be afraid to experiment – find out what type of music works best for you.

We hope you enjoy our Volume 2, 4th edition as much as we enjoyed putting it together.

JoAnn Zerwekh

Jo Carol Claborn

TABLE OF CONTENTS

Basic Care

Assessment

Fluids, Acid-Base and Electrolytes

Pharmacology

Psychosocial

Immune

Sensory

Hematology

Endocrine

Respiratory

Cardiac

© 2012 Nursing Education Consultants, Inc.

Reproductive

Integumentary

Vascular

Maternity and Newborn

© 2012 Nursing Education
Consultants, Inc.

ACTIVITIES OF DAILY LIVING

ADLs = BATTED
(Activities of Daily Living)

Bathing

Ambulation

Toileting

Transfers

Eating

Dressing

INSTRUMENTAL ACTIVITIES OF DAILY LIVING

IADLs = 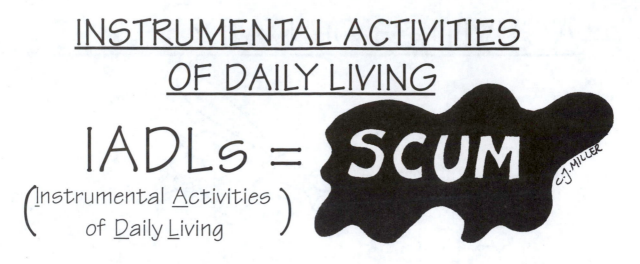 **SCUM**

(**I**nstrumental **A**ctivities of **D**aily **L**iving)

C.J. MILLER

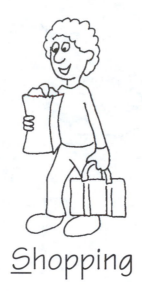

Shopping

Cooking / **C**leaning

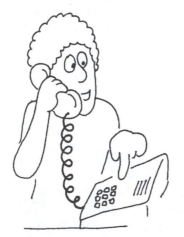

Using Telephone or Transportation

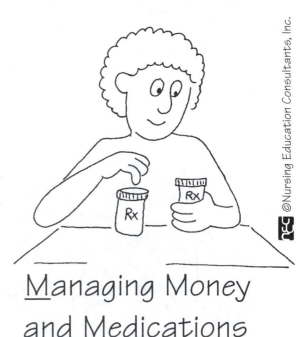

Managing Money and Medications

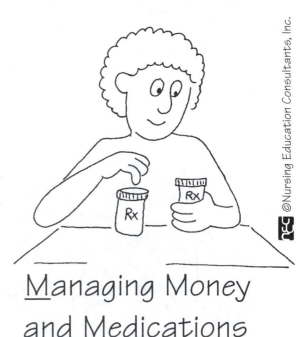

FOUR Cs OF INITIAL DIRECTION

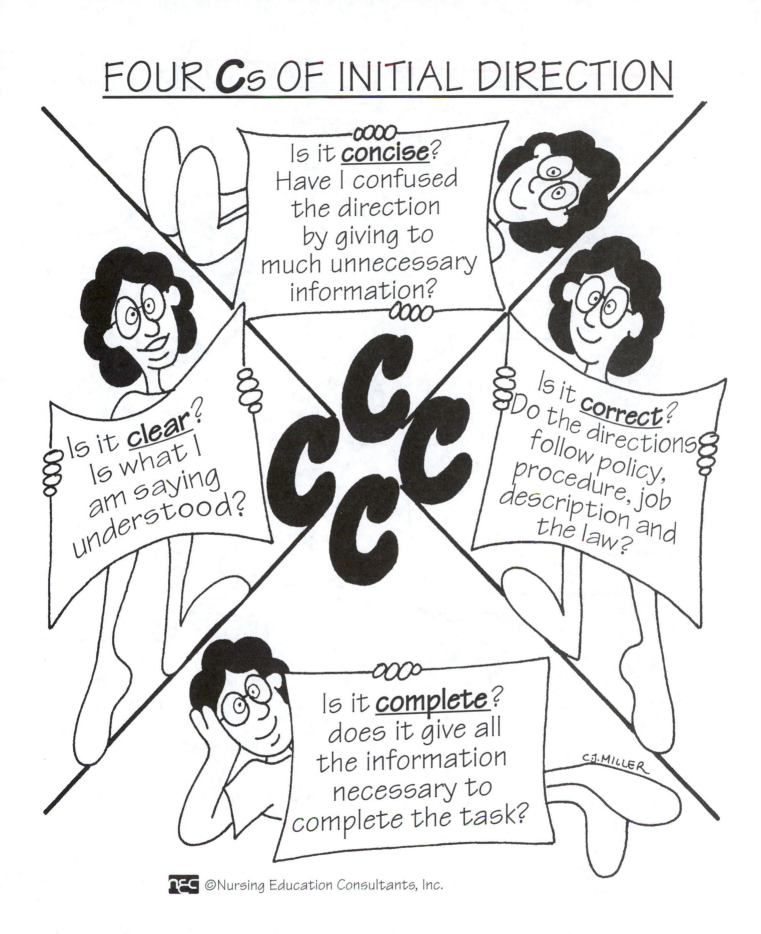

Is it **concise**? Have I confused the direction by giving to much unnecessary information?

Is it **clear**? Is what I am saying understood?

Is it **correct**? Do the directions follow policy, procedure, job description and the law?

Is it **complete**? does it give all the information necessary to complete the task?

C.J. MILLER

BLEEDING PRECAUTIONS

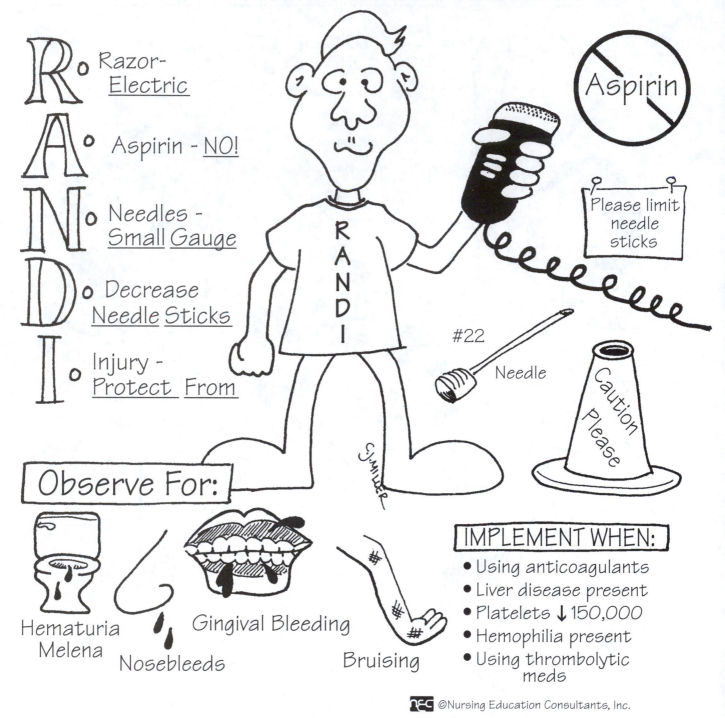

R - Razor- Electric

A - Aspirin - NO!

N - Needles - Small Gauge

D - Decrease Needle Sticks

I - Injury - Protect From

Aspirin

Please limit needle sticks

#22 Needle

Caution Please

Observe For:

Hematuria Melena

Nosebleeds

Gingival Bleeding

Bruising

IMPLEMENT WHEN:

- Using anticoagulants
- Liver disease present
- Platelets ↓ 150,000
- Hemophilia present
- Using thrombolytic meds

©Nursing Education Consultants, Inc.

Basic Care
NursingEd.com

BLOOD PRESSURE

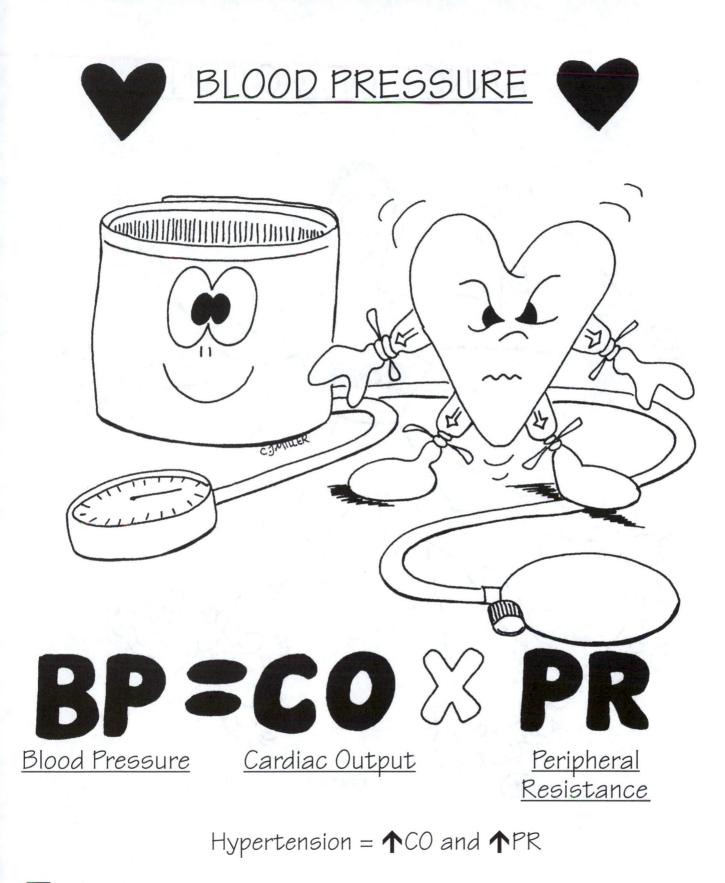

BP = CO X PR

Blood Pressure   Cardiac Output   Peripheral Resistance

Hypertension = ↑CO and ↑PR

RANGE OF MOTION

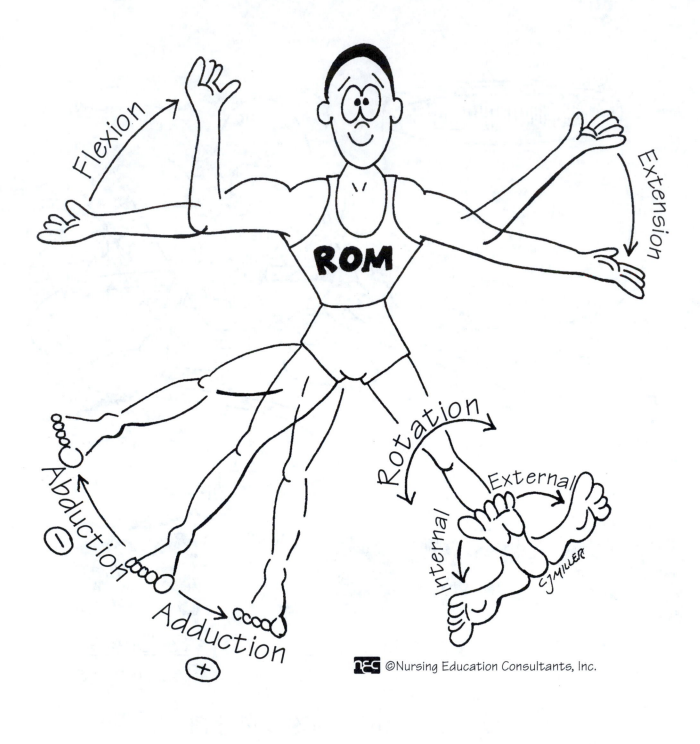

ROM

Flexion

Extension

Abduction

Adduction

Rotation

Internal

External

CJ MILLER

Basic Care
NursingEd.com

© 2012 Nursing Education
Consultants, Inc.

CANES AND WALKERS

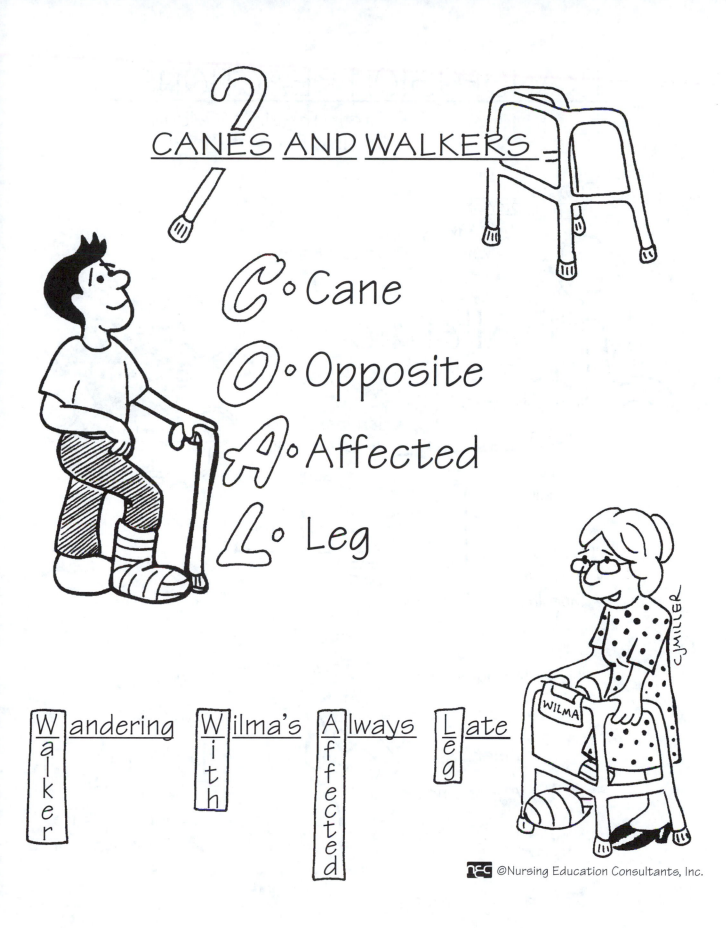

C ◦ Cane

O ◦ Opposite

A ◦ Affected

L ◦ Leg

Wandering **W**ilma's **A**lways **L**ate
alker **i**th **f**fected **e**g
l **t** **f** **g**
k **h** **e**
e **c**
r **t**
e
d

TRANSFUSION REACTIONS:

(Occurs In The First 10-15 Min)
Or First 50cc of Blood

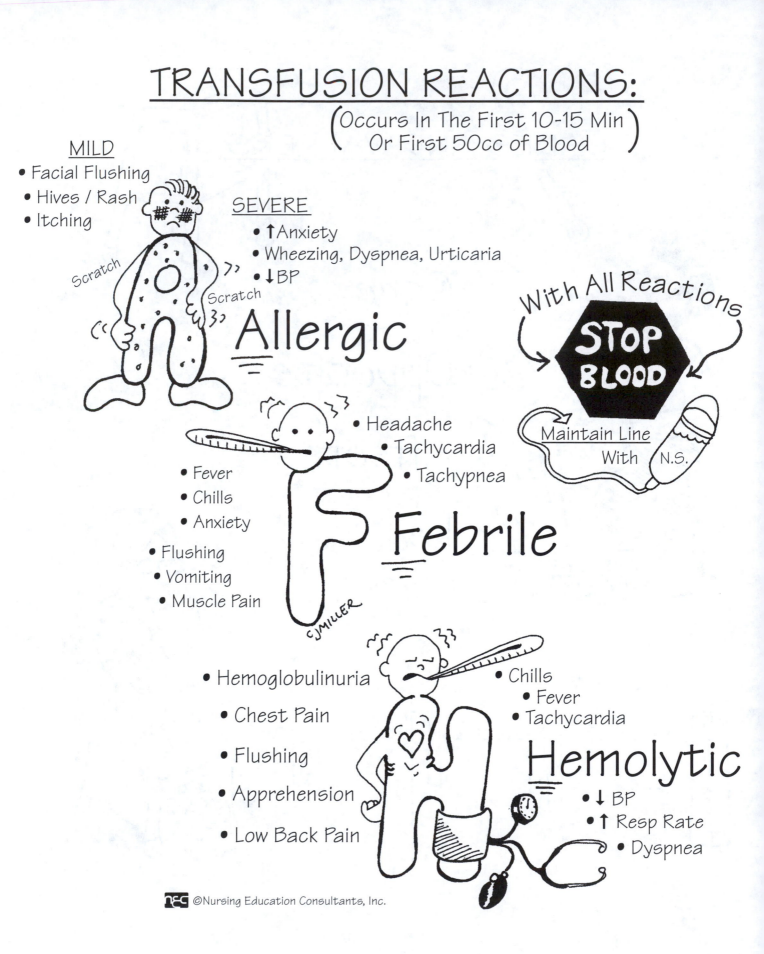

MILD
- Facial Flushing
- Hives / Rash
- Itching

Scratch
Scratch

SEVERE
- ↑Anxiety
- Wheezing, Dyspnea, Urticaria
- ↓BP

Allergic

With All Reactions

STOP BLOOD

Maintain Line
With N.S.

- Headache
- Tachycardia
- Tachypnea

- Fever
- Chills
- Anxiety
- Flushing
- Vomiting
- Muscle Pain

Febrile

CJMILLER

- Hemoglobulinuria
- Chest Pain
- Flushing
- Apprehension
- Low Back Pain

- Chills
- Fever
- Tachycardia

Hemolytic

- ↓ BP
- ↑ Resp Rate
- Dyspnea

TYPES of EXUDATE

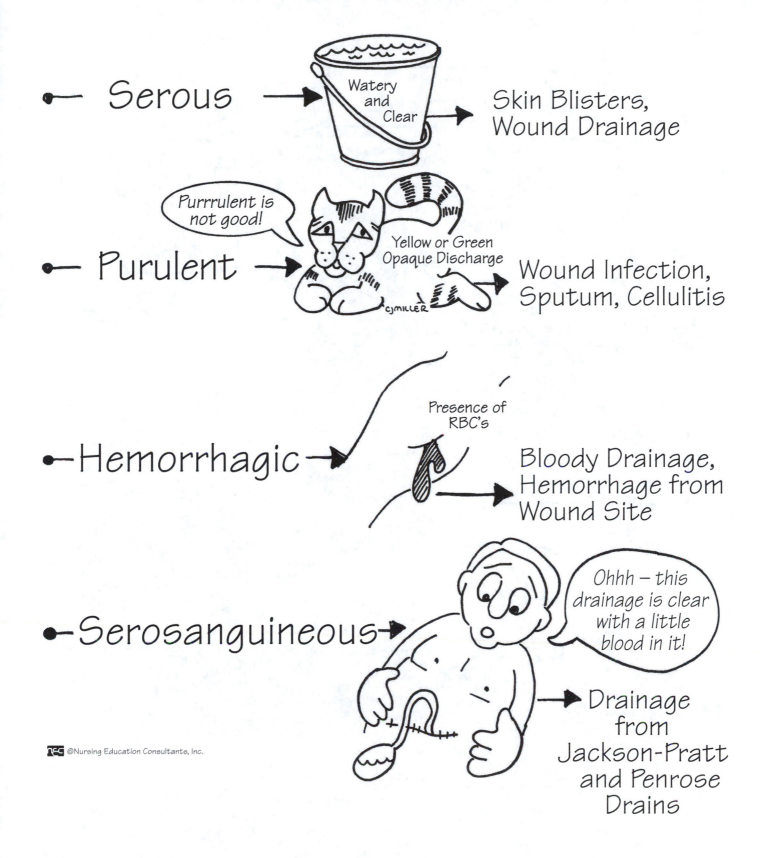

Serous → Watery and Clear → Skin Blisters, Wound Drainage

Purulent → *Purrrulent is not good!* Yellow or Green Opaque Discharge → Wound Infection, Sputum, Cellulitis

Hemorrhagic → Presence of RBC's → Bloody Drainage, Hemorrhage from Wound Site

Serosanguineous → *Ohhh — this drainage is clear with a little blood in it!* → Drainage from Jackson-Pratt and Penrose Drains

IMMUNE SYSTEM RESPONSE

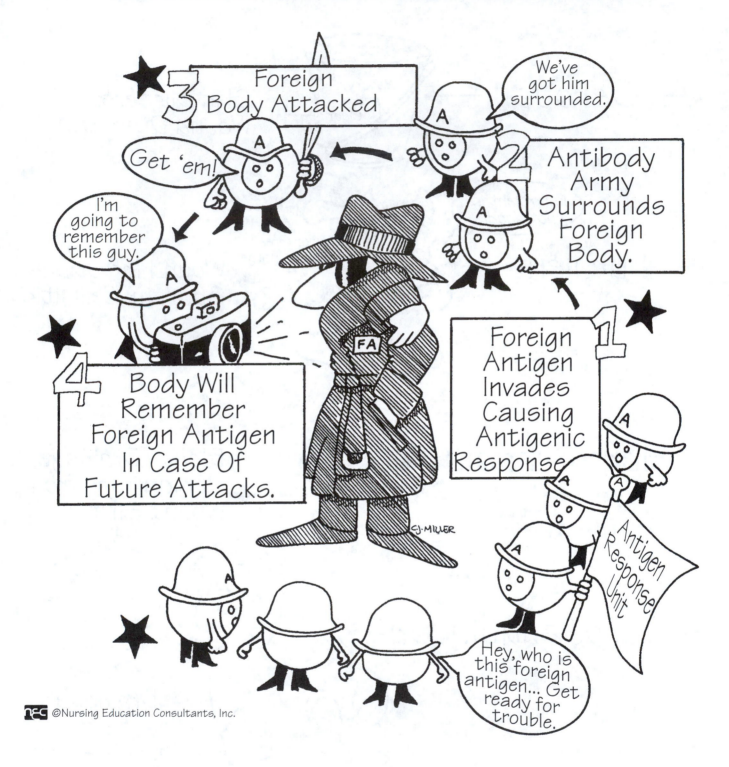

ANALGESIA vs ANESTHESIA

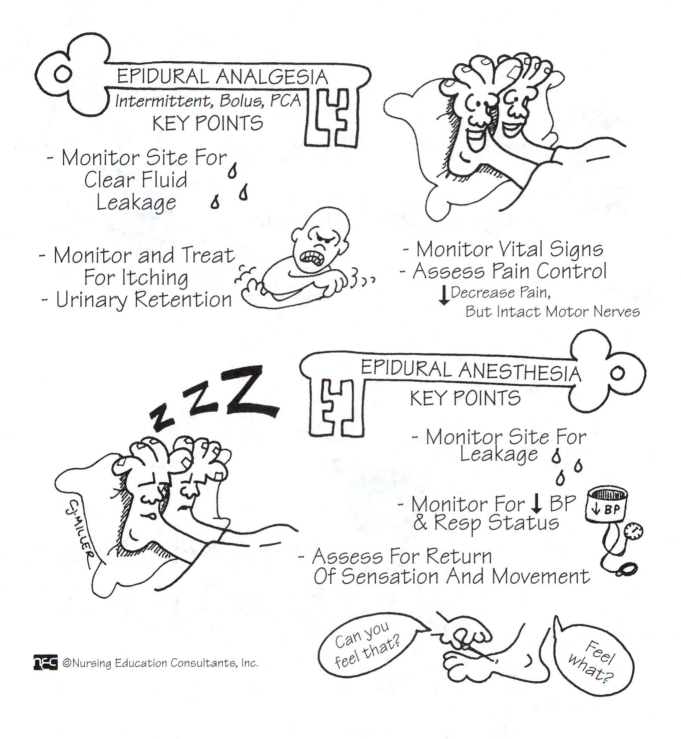

EPIDURAL ANALGESIA
Intermittent, Bolus, PCA
KEY POINTS

- Monitor Site For Clear Fluid Leakage

- Monitor and Treat For Itching
- Urinary Retention

- Monitor Vital Signs
- Assess Pain Control
  ↓ Decrease Pain, But Intact Motor Nerves

EPIDURAL ANESTHESIA
KEY POINTS

- Monitor Site For Leakage

- Monitor For ↓ BP & Resp Status

- Assess For Return Of Sensation And Movement

Can you feel that?

Feel what?

"AUTONOMIC NERVOUS SYSTEM RESPONSE"

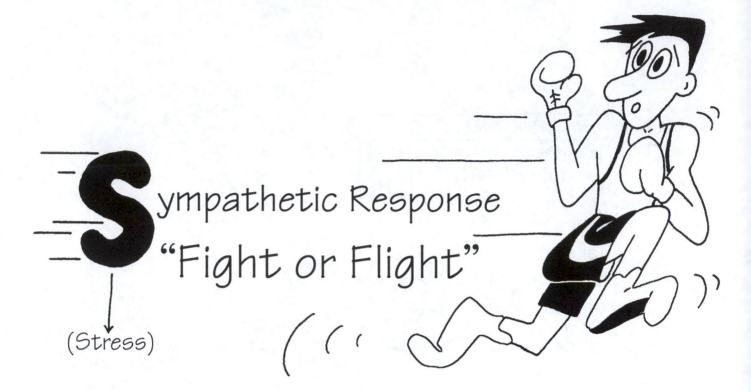

Sympathetic Response
"Fight or Flight"

(Stress)

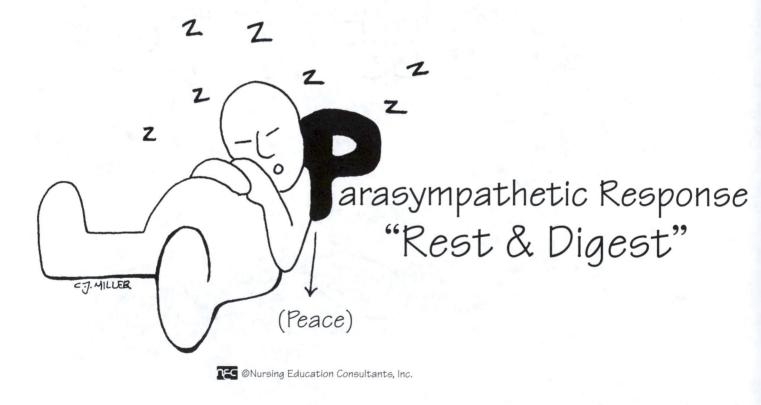

Parasympathetic Response
"Rest & Digest"

(Peace)

Basic Care
NursingEd.com

IS IT A COLD OR THE FLU?

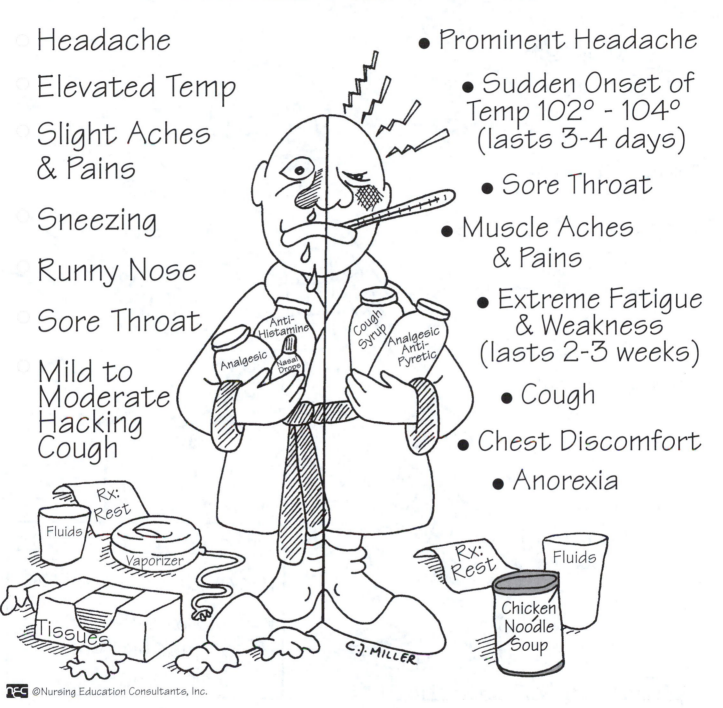

- Headache
- Elevated Temp
- Slight Aches & Pains
- Sneezing
- Runny Nose
- Sore Throat
- Mild to Moderate Hacking Cough

- Prominent Headache
- Sudden Onset of Temp 102° - 104° (lasts 3-4 days)
- Sore Throat
- Muscle Aches & Pains
- Extreme Fatigue & Weakness (lasts 2-3 weeks)
- Cough
- Chest Discomfort
- Anorexia

SPECIAL CONSIDERATIONS FOR OLDER ADULTS

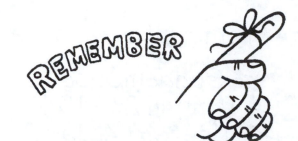

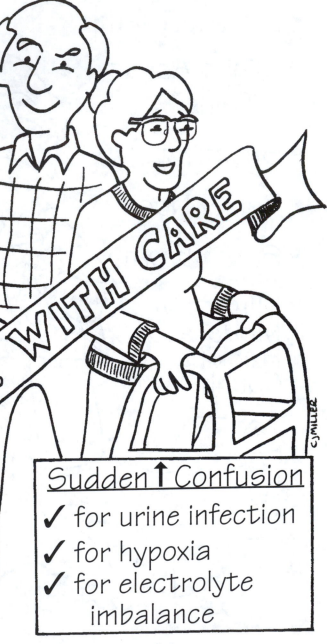

↓ Tolerance to Meds
(Prevent Over Sedation)

↓ IV Rate to Avoid Fluid Overload

↑ Risk Of:

- Respiratory Depression
- Pneumonia
- Disorientation
- Skin Breakdown
- Problems with:
  Circulation
  Nutrition
  Constipation
  Fluid & Electrolyte
    Balance
- ↑ Balance and
    ↓ Falls

Sudden ↑ Confusion

✓ for urine infection
✓ for hypoxia
✓ for electrolyte
    imbalance

☆Clinical Management☆

Treat coexisting medical disorders
   Cardiac problems
   Peripheral vascular disease
   Neurological disorders

 ©Nursing Education Consultants, Inc.

NORMAL ELIMINATION

PROMOTE ELIMINATION

P Position - Upright, sitting
O Output - Adequate hydration
O Offer Fluids
P Privacy
E Exercise
R Report Results

OBSERVE

S Size (Amount)
C Consistency
O Occult Blood
O Odor
P Peristalsis

©Nursing Education Consultants, Inc.

HEAT and COLD APPLICATIONS

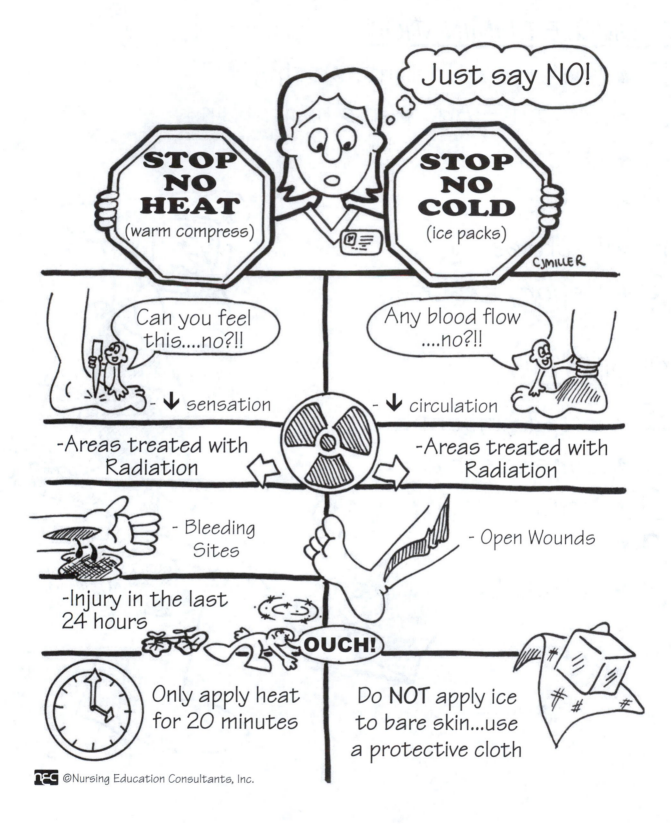

HAND HYGIENE

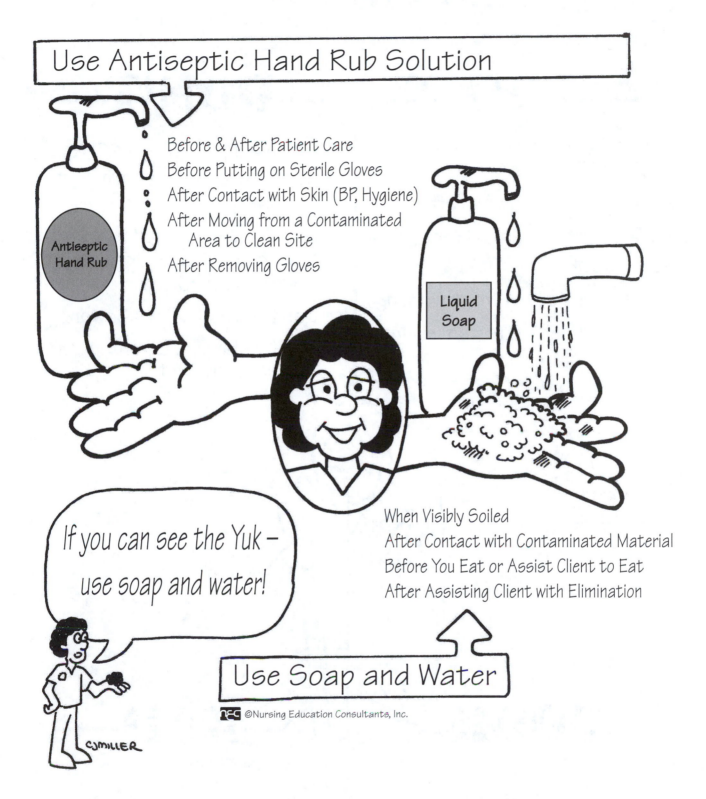

Use Antiseptic Hand Rub Solution

Before & After Patient Care
Before Putting on Sterile Gloves
After Contact with Skin (BP, Hygiene)
After Moving from a Contaminated
    Area to Clean Site
After Removing Gloves

Antiseptic
Hand Rub

Liquid
Soap

If you can see the Yuk –
use soap and water!

When Visibly Soiled
After Contact with Contaminated Material
Before You Eat or Assist Client to Eat
After Assisting Client with Elimination

Use Soap and Water

©Nursing Education Consultants, Inc.

CJMILLER

Basic Care
NursingEd.com

INFORMATICS

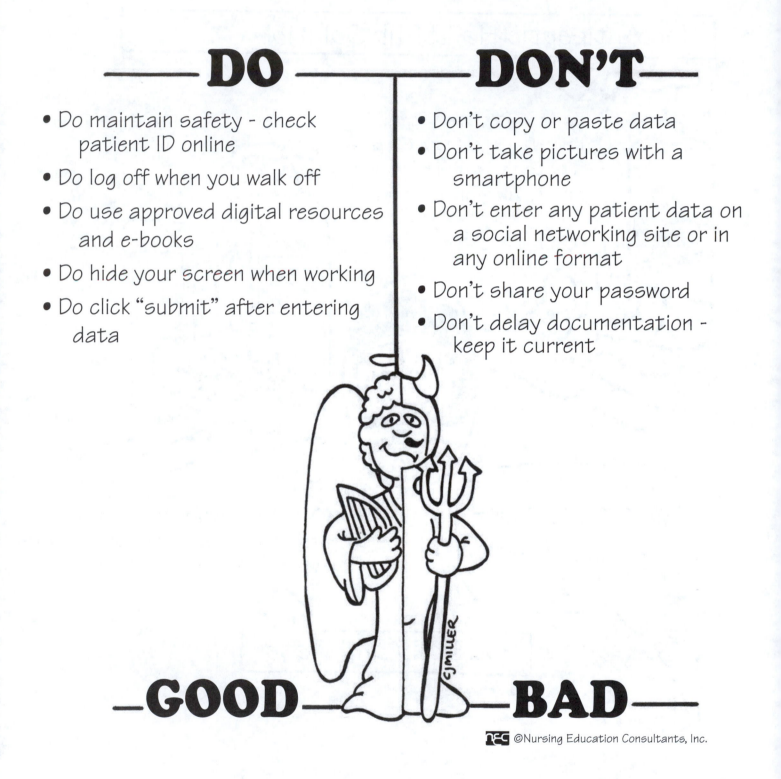

— DO —

- Do maintain safety - check patient ID online
- Do log off when you walk off
- Do use approved digital resources and e-books
- Do hide your screen when working
- Do click "submit" after entering data

—DON'T—

- Don't copy or paste data
- Don't take pictures with a smartphone
- Don't enter any patient data on a social networking site or in any online format
- Don't share your password
- Don't delay documentation - keep it current

—GOOD

BAD—

©Nursing Education Consultants, Inc.

Basic Care
NursingEd.com

© 2012 Nursing Education
Consultants, Inc.

TOOLS OF PHYSICAL ASSESSMENT

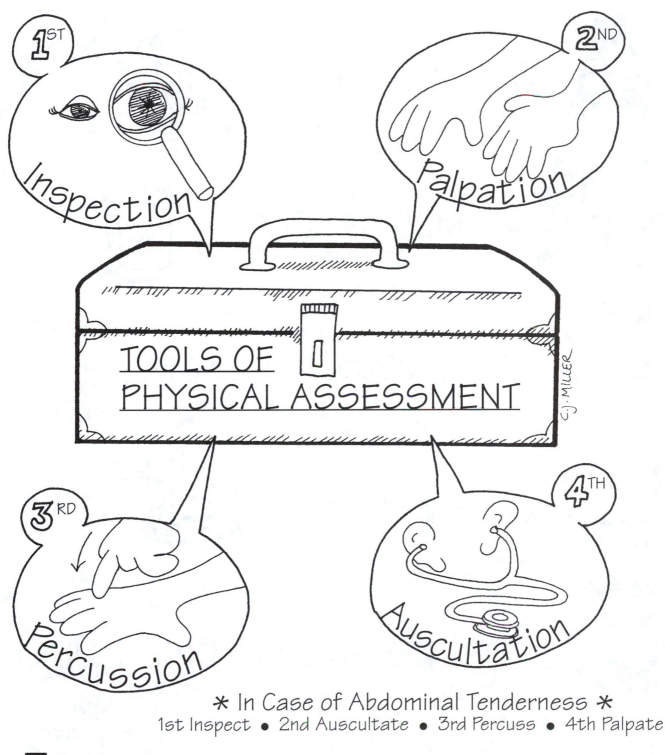

* In Case of Abdominal Tenderness *
1st Inspect • 2nd Auscultate • 3rd Percuss • 4th Palpate

©Nursing Education Consultants, Inc.

TRAUMA SURVEY (AFTER INITIAL ASSESSMENT)

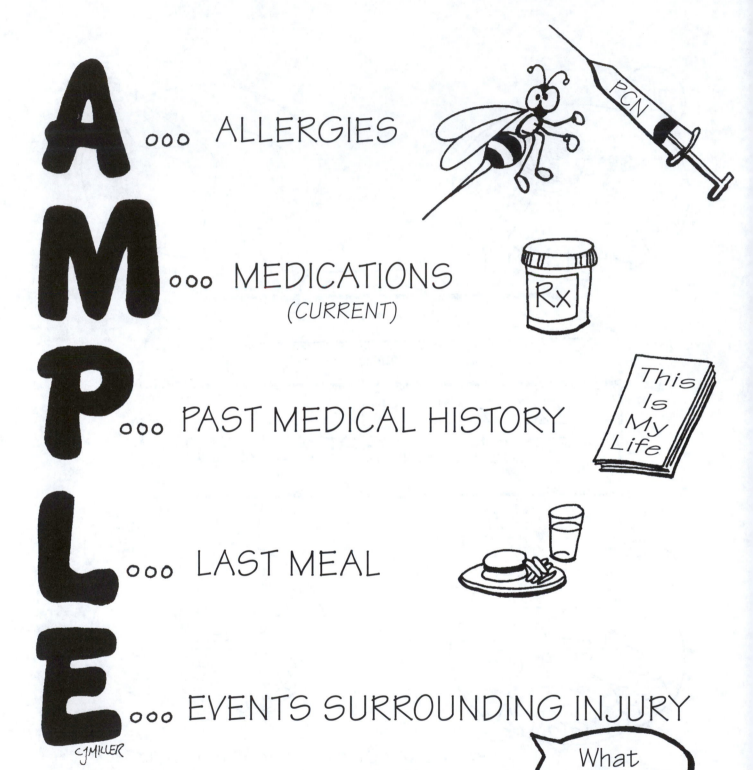

A ... ALLERGIES

M ... MEDICATIONS (CURRENT)

P ... PAST MEDICAL HISTORY

L ... LAST MEAL

E ... EVENTS SURROUNDING INJURY

6-Ps OF DYSPNEA

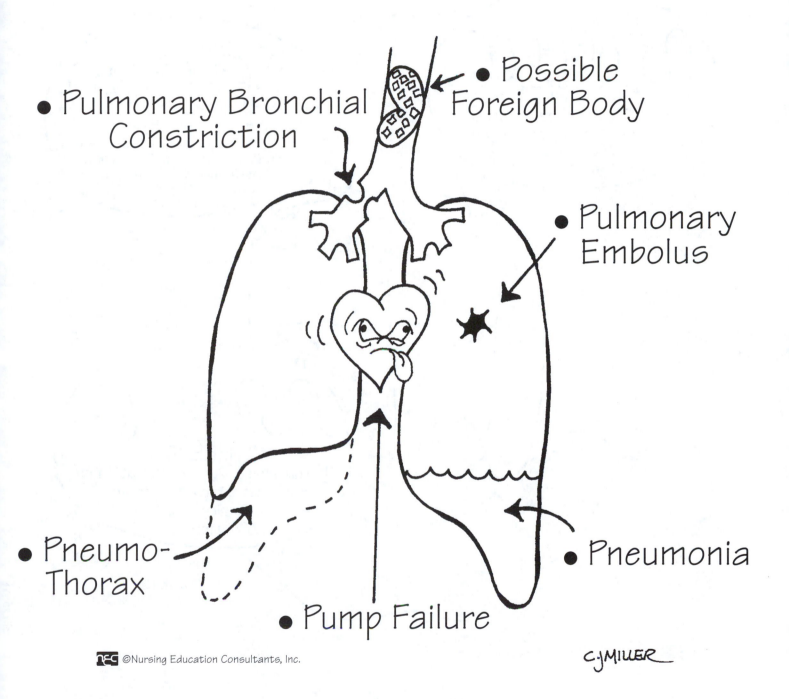

- Pulmonary Bronchial Constriction
- Possible Foreign Body
- Pulmonary Embolus
- Pneumo-Thorax
- Pneumonia
- Pump Failure

C.J MILLER

LUNG SOUNDS

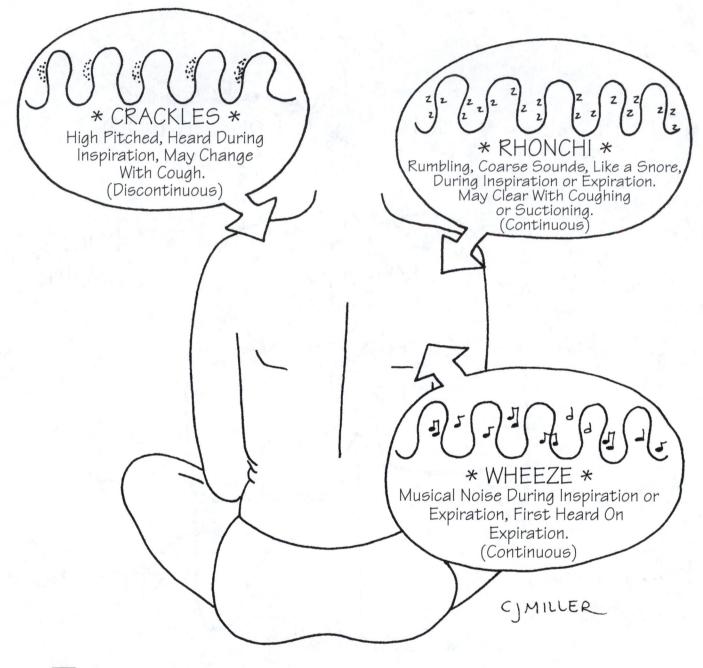

* CRACKLES *
High Pitched, Heard During
Inspiration, May Change
With Cough.
(Discontinuous)

* RHONCHI *
Rumbling, Coarse Sounds, Like a Snore,
During Inspiration or Expiration.
May Clear With Coughing
or Suctioning.
(Continuous)

* WHEEZE *
Musical Noise During Inspiration or
Expiration, First Heard On
Expiration.
(Continuous)

CJ MILLER

REASONS FOR UNCONSCIOUSNESS
(SKIN COLOR)

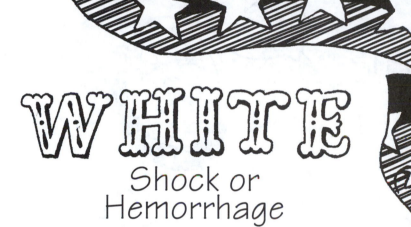

RED
Stroke or ↑ BP

WHITE
Shock or
Hemorrhage

BLUE
Respiratory
or
Cardiac Arrest

S.J. MILLER

LEVELS OF CONSCIOUSNESS

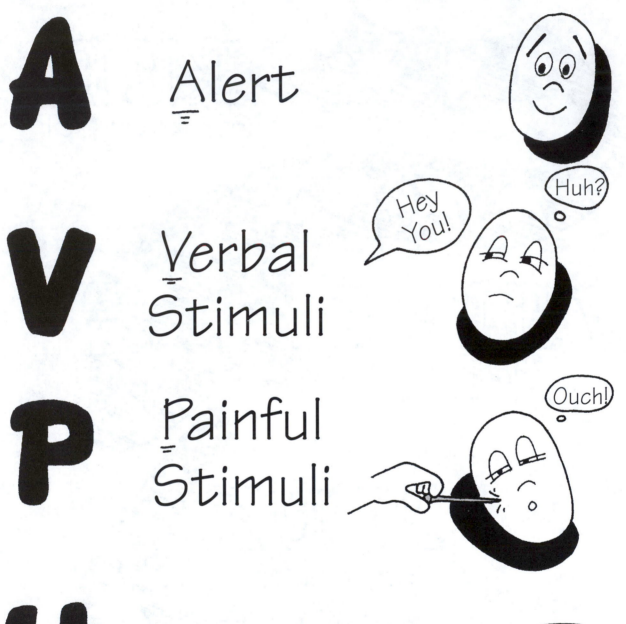

A Alert

V Verbal Stimuli

P Painful Stimuli

U Unresponsive

©Nursing Education Consultants, Inc.

Assessment
NursingEd.com

© 2012 Nursing Education
Consultants, Inc.

SHOCK

SHOCK IT TO ME, BABY...

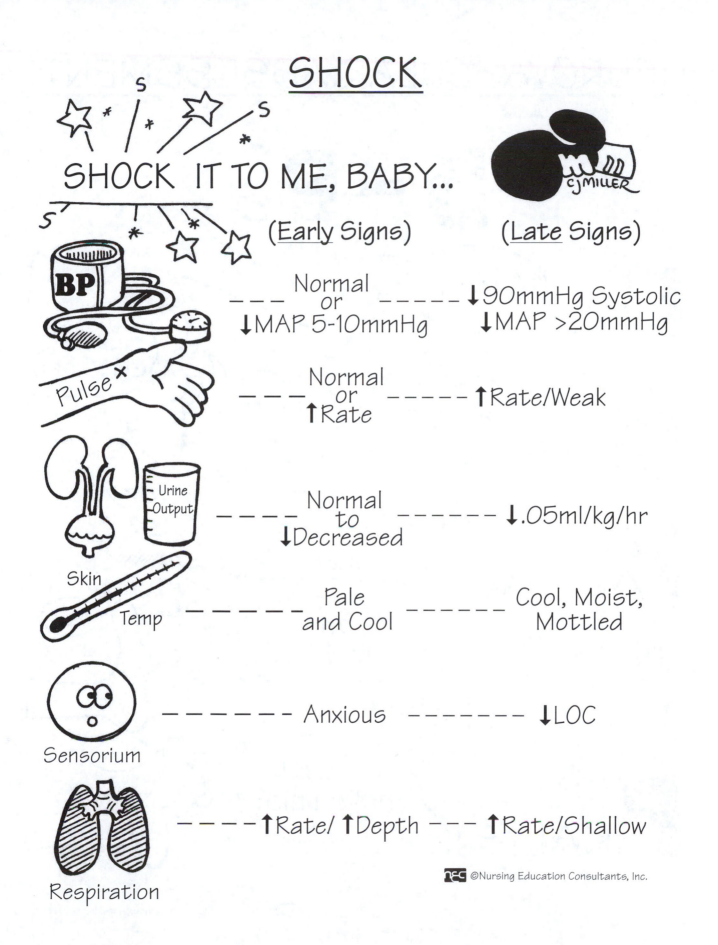

	(Early Signs)	(Late Signs)
BP	Normal or ↓MAP 5-10mmHg	↓90mmHg Systolic ↓MAP >20mmHg
Pulse	Normal or ↑Rate	↑Rate/Weak
Urine Output	Normal to ↓Decreased	↓.05ml/kg/hr
Skin Temp	Pale and Cool	Cool, Moist, Mottled
Sensorium	Anxious	↓LOC
Respiration	↑Rate/ ↑Depth	↑Rate/Shallow

NEUROVASCULAR ASSESSMENT

5-Ps

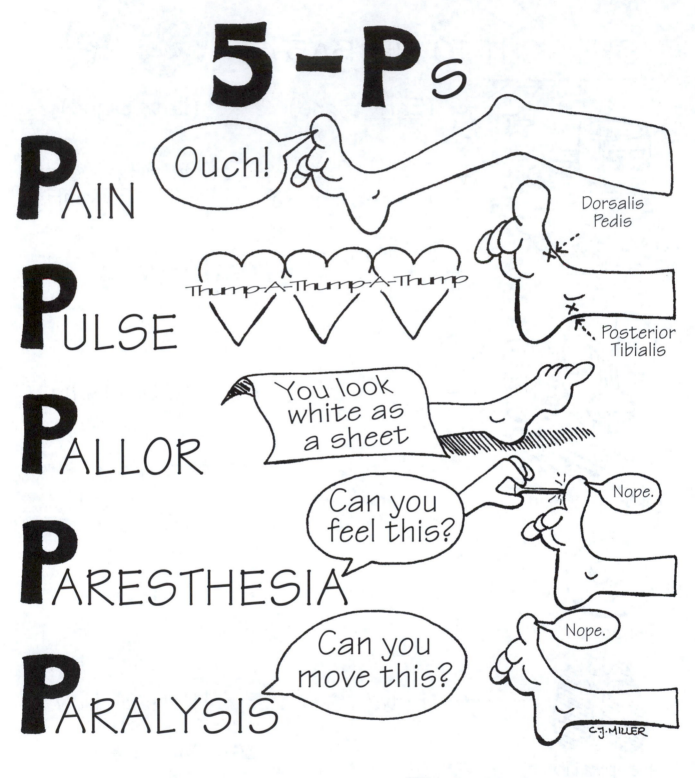

PAIN

PULSE

PALLOR

PARESTHESIA

PARALYSIS

Assessment
NursingEd.com

© 2012 Nursing Education
Consultants, Inc.

5 AREAS FOR LISTENING TO THE HEART

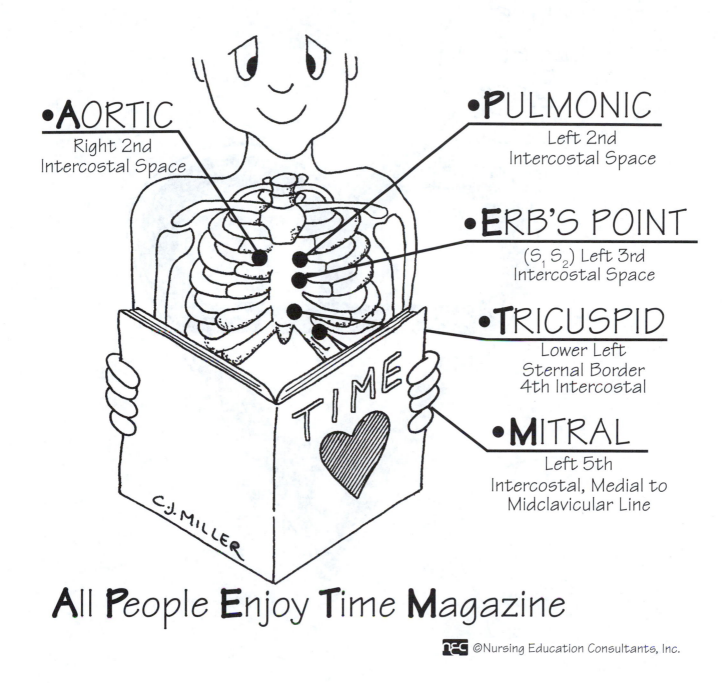

•AORTIC
Right 2nd
Intercostal Space

•PULMONIC
Left 2nd
Intercostal Space

•ERB'S POINT
$(S_1 S_2)$ Left 3rd
Intercostal Space

•TRICUSPID
Lower Left
Sternal Border
4th Intercostal

•MITRAL
Left 5th
Intercostal, Medial to
Midclavicular Line

C.J. MILLER

TIME

All People Enjoy Time Magazine

©Nursing Education Consultants, Inc.

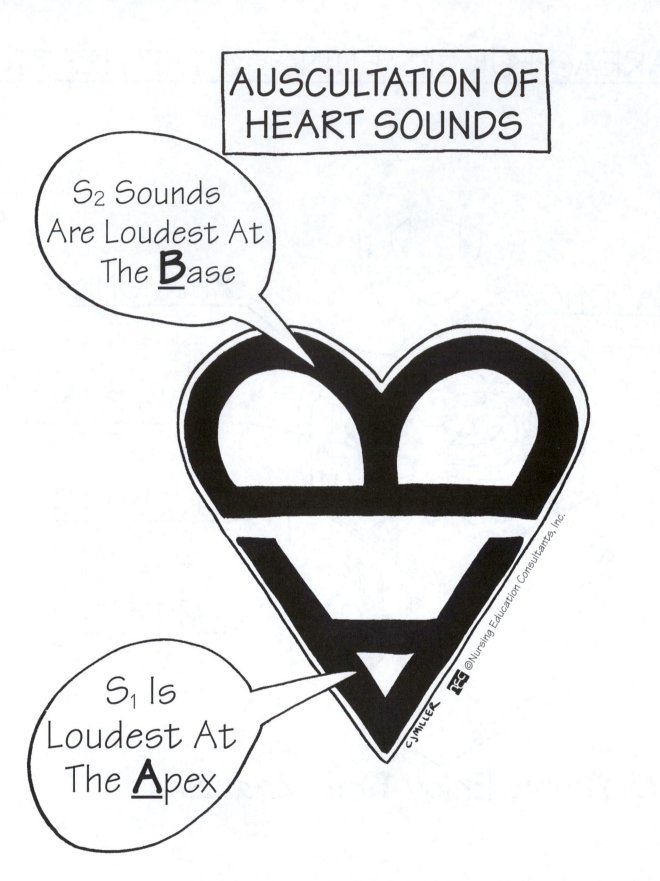

PMI - 5th Intercostal Space, Left Midclavicular Line

Assessment
NursingEd.com

© 2012 Nursing Education
Consultants, Inc.

HEART SOUNDS

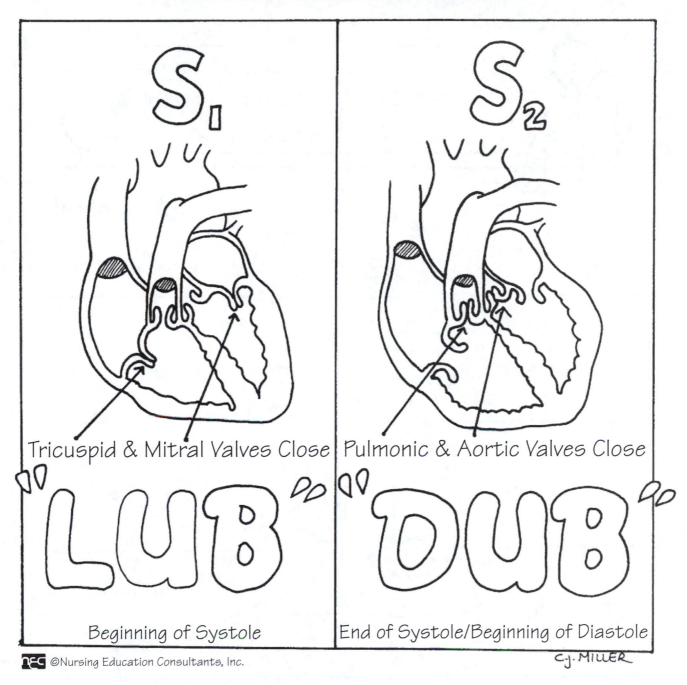

S_1

S_2

Tricuspid & Mitral Valves Close   Pulmonic & Aortic Valves Close

"LUB"   "DUB"

Beginning of Systole   End of Systole/Beginning of Diastole

C.J. MILLER

PRIORITIZATION and DELEGATION

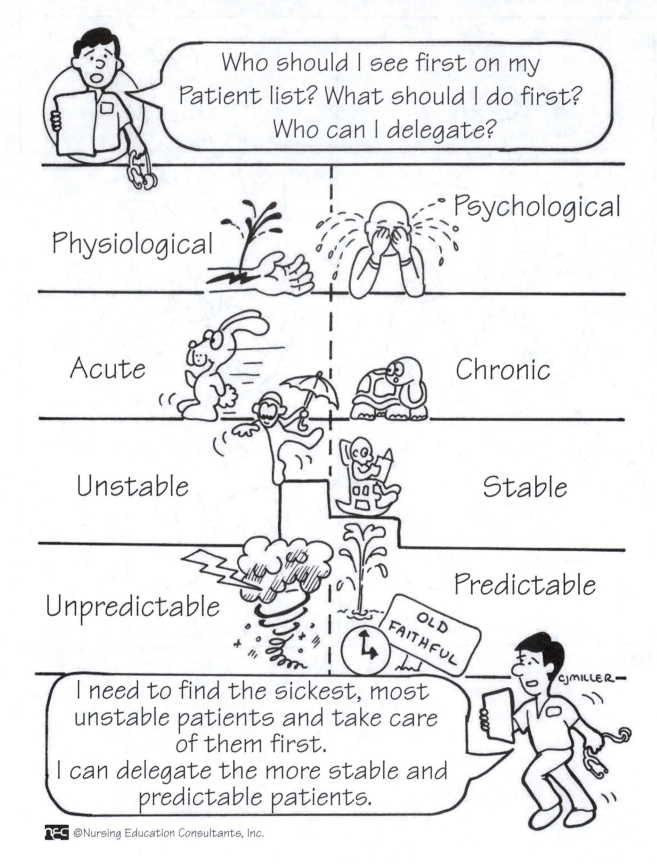

Who should I see first on my Patient list? What should I do first? Who can I delegate?

Physiological

Psychological

Acute

Chronic

Unstable

Stable

Unpredictable

Predictable

OLD FAITHFUL

I need to find the sickest, most unstable patients and take care of them first.
I can delegate the more stable and predictable patients.

Assessment
NursingEd.com

© 2012 Nursing Education Consultants, Inc.

BASICS OF HYDRATION

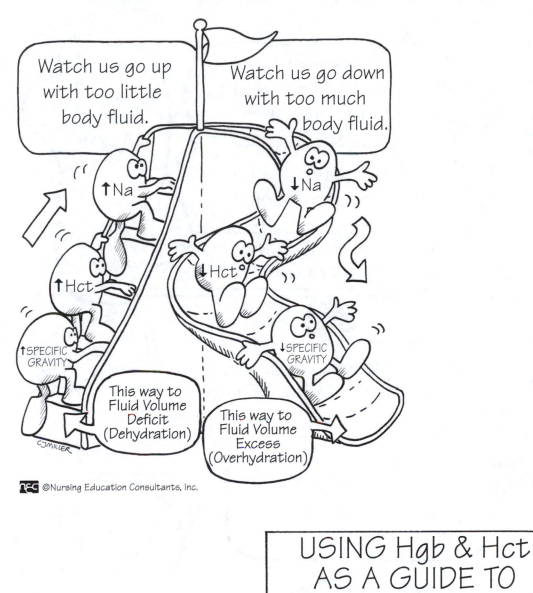

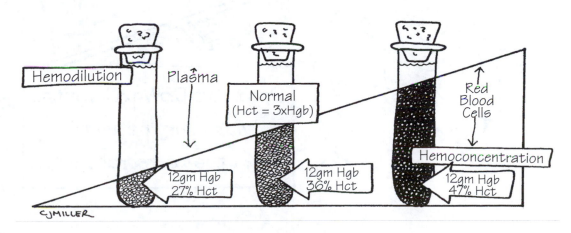

TOP 5 FLUIDS

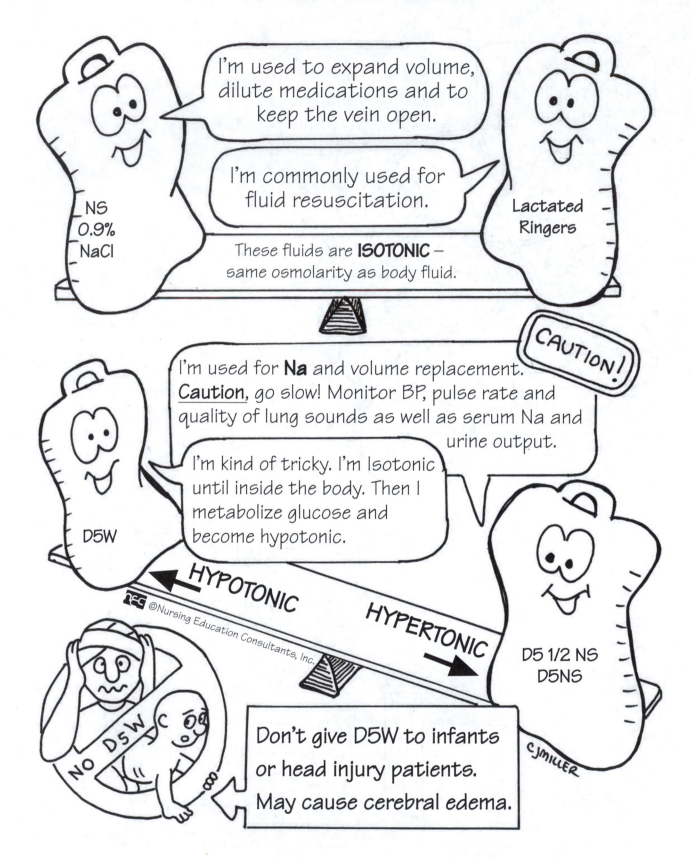

I'm used to expand volume, dilute medications and to keep the vein open.

I'm commonly used for fluid resuscitation.

NS 0.9% NaCl

Lactated Ringers

These fluids are **ISOTONIC** – same osmolarity as body fluid.

CAUTION!

I'm used for **Na** and volume replacement. <u>Caution</u>, go slow! Monitor BP, pulse rate and quality of lung sounds as well as serum Na and urine output.

I'm kind of tricky. I'm Isotonic until inside the body. Then I metabolize glucose and become hypotonic.

D5W

HYPOTONIC

HYPERTONIC

D5 1/2 NS D5NS

©Nursing Education Consultants, Inc.

CJMILLER

NO D5W

Don't give D5W to infants or head injury patients. May cause cerebral edema.

Fluid Balance, Acid-Base and Electrolytes
NursingEd.com

ACIDOSIS - ALKALOSIS

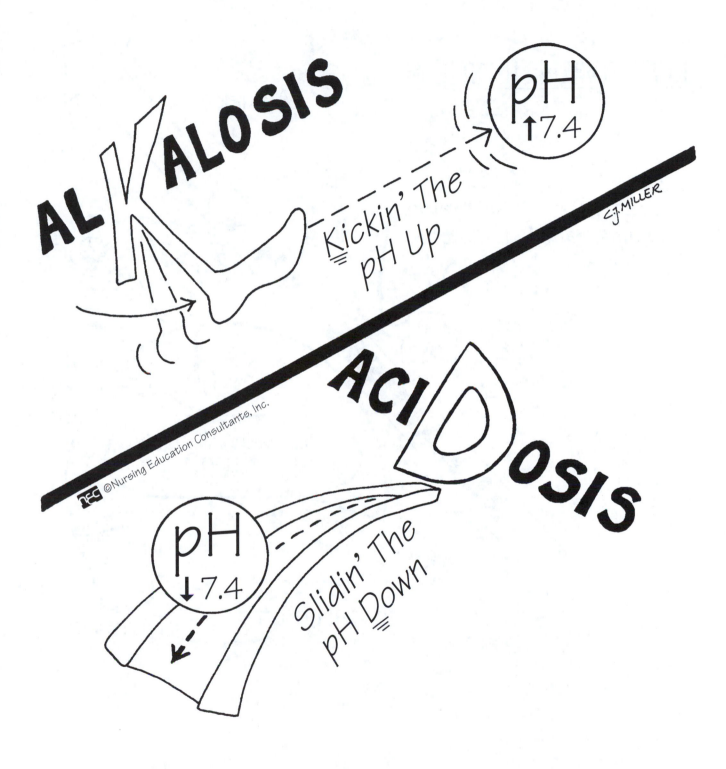

ALKALOSIS

Kickin' The pH Up

pH ↑7.4

ACIDOSIS

pH ↓7.4

Slidin' The pH Down

C.J. MILLER

©Nursing Education Consultants, Inc.

CAUSES OF ALKALOSIS

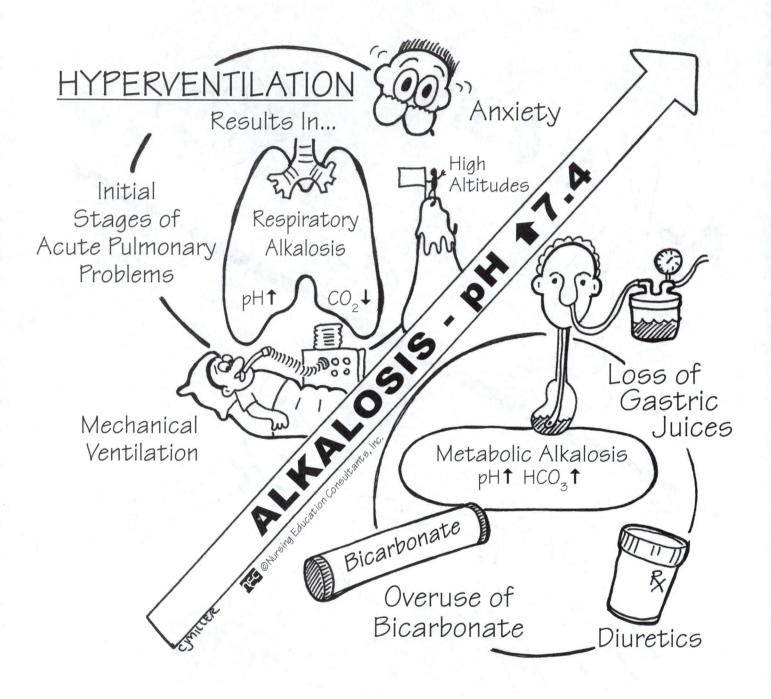

HYPERVENTILATION

Results In...

Anxiety

High Altitudes

Initial Stages of Acute Pulmonary Problems

Respiratory Alkalosis

$pH \uparrow$ $CO_2 \downarrow$

ALKALOSIS - pH $\uparrow$ 7.4

Mechanical Ventilation

Loss of Gastric Juices

Metabolic Alkalosis
$pH \uparrow$ $HCO_3 \uparrow$

Bicarbonate

Overuse of Bicarbonate

Diuretics

©Nursing Education Consultants, Inc.

Fluid Balance, Acid-Base and Electrolytes
NursingEd.com

CAUSES OF ACIDOSIS

HYPOVENTILATION
Results in...

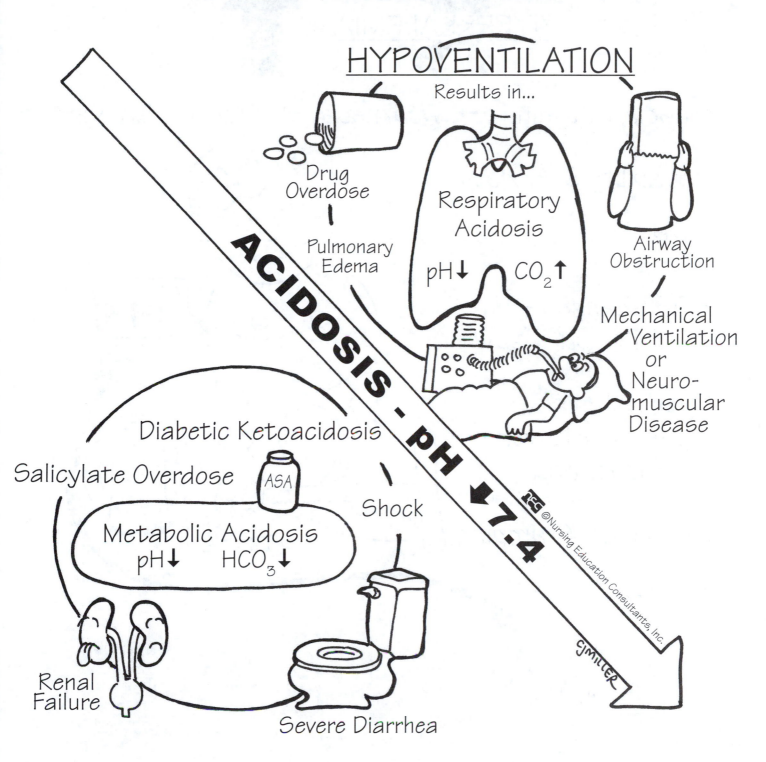

Drug Overdose

Pulmonary Edema

Respiratory Acidosis

$pH\downarrow$ $CO_2\uparrow$

Airway Obstruction

Mechanical Ventilation or Neuro-muscular Disease

ACIDOSIS - pH ◄ 7.4

Diabetic Ketoacidosis

Salicylate Overdose

ASA

Metabolic Acidosis
$pH\downarrow$ $HCO_3\downarrow$

Shock

Renal Failure

Severe Diarrhea

©Nursing Education Consultants, Inc.

Fluid Balance, Acid-Base and Electrolytes
NursingEd.com

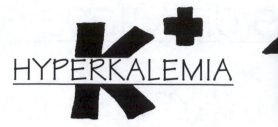

HYPERKALEMIA

* Muscle Twitching → Weakness → Flaccid Paralysis

* Irritability & Anxiety

* ↓ BP

* ECG Changes -
    Tall Peaked T Waves

* Dysrhythmias -
    Irregular Rhythm
    Bradycardia

* Abdominal Cramping

* Diarrhea

Urine Output

CJMILLER

Flat P   Wide QRS
    Peaked T
Prolonged P-R

©Nursing Education Consultants, Inc.

Fluid Balance, Acid-Base and Electrolytes
NursingEd.com

POTASSIUM DEFICIT

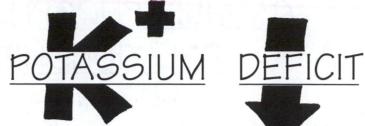

* **A**lkalosis

* **S**hallow Respirations

* **I**rritability

* **C**onfusion, Drowsiness

* **W**eakness, Fatigue

* **A**rrhythmias -
    Tachycardia
    Irregular Rhythm and/or
    Bradycardia

* **L**ethargy

* **T**hready Pulse

* ↓ Intestinal Motility
    Nausea
    Vomiting
    Ileus

I am a SIC WALT.

Wake us up when it's over

ACME CO.

©Nursing Education Consultants, Inc.

CALCIUM-PHOSPHORUS RELATIONSHIP

- The Ups and Down -

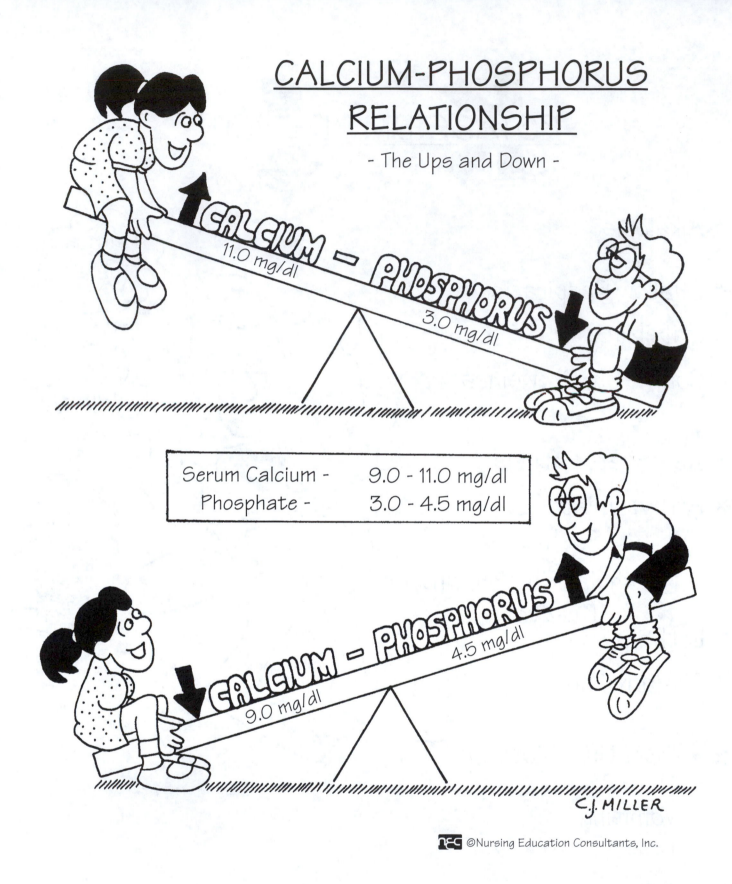

Serum Calcium - 9.0 - 11.0 mg/dl
Phosphate - 3.0 - 4.5 mg/dl

C.J. MILLER

©Nursing Education Consultants, Inc.

Fluid Balance, Acid-Base and Electrolytes
NursingEd.com

© 2012 Nursing Education
Consultants, Inc.

HEAT EXHAUSTION

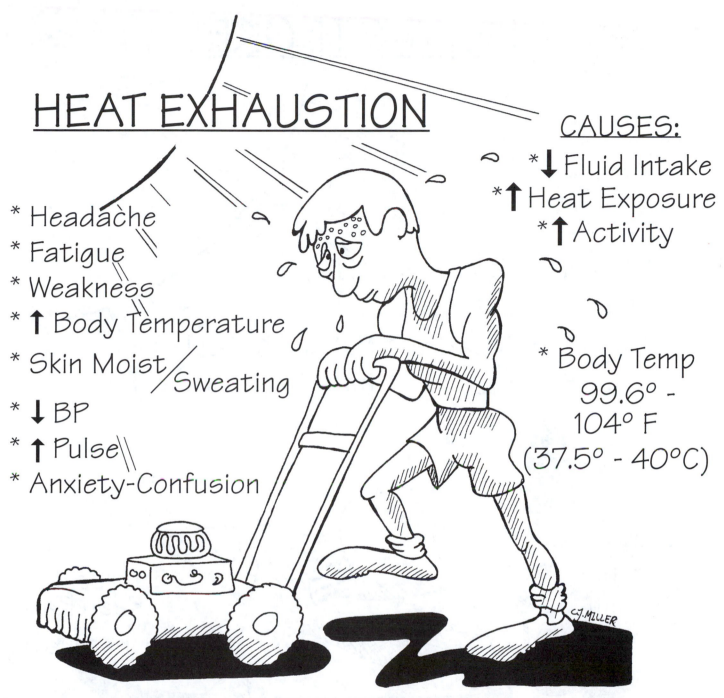

* Headache
* Fatigue
* Weakness
* ↑ Body Temperature
* Skin Moist / Sweating
* ↓ BP
* ↑ Pulse
* Anxiety-Confusion

CAUSES:
* ↓ Fluid Intake
* ↑ Heat Exposure
* ↑ Activity

* Body Temp 99.6° - 104° F (37.5° - 40°C)

(Management - Cool Down, Oral Rehydrating Solutions, Rest)

HEAT STROKE

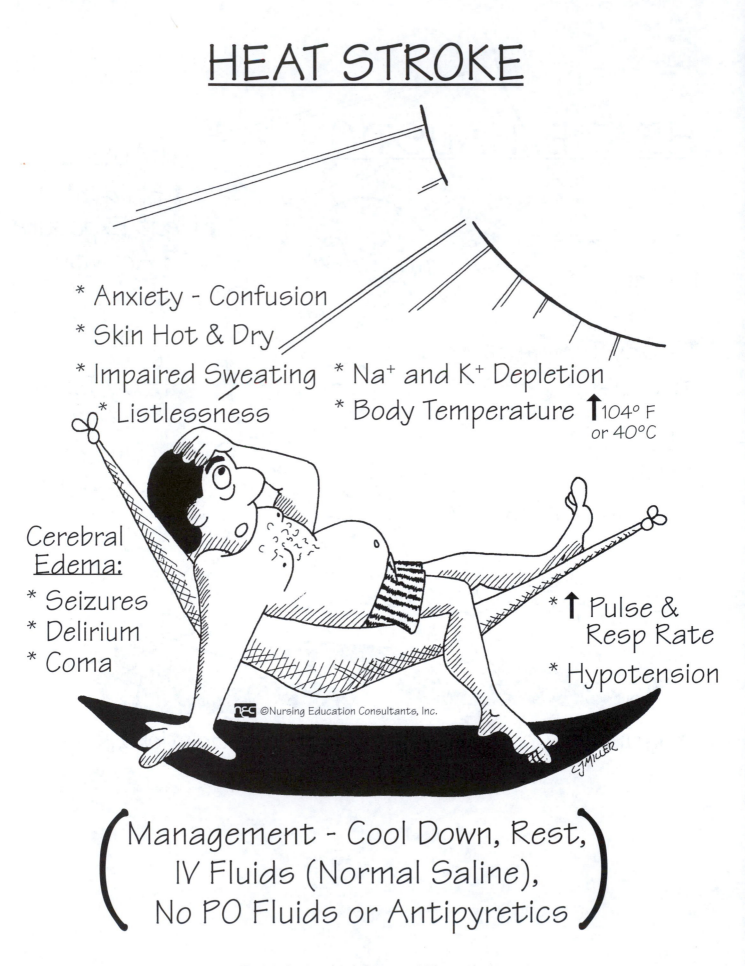

* Anxiety - Confusion
* Skin Hot & Dry
* Impaired Sweating
* Listlessness

* Na^+ and K^+ Depletion
* Body Temperature ↑104° F or 40°C

Cerebral Edema:
* Seizures
* Delirium
* Coma

* ↑ Pulse & Resp Rate
* Hypotension

©Nursing Education Consultants, Inc.

(Management - Cool Down, Rest, IV Fluids (Normal Saline), No PO Fluids or Antipyretics)

Fluid Balance, Acid-Base and Electrolytes
NursingEd.com

ADMINISTRATION OF MEDICATIONS BY INHALATION

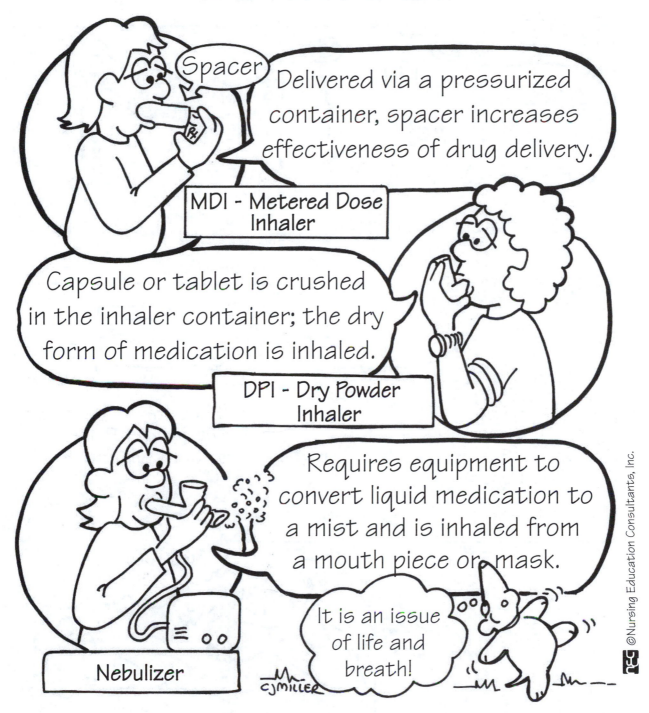

TRANSDERMAL MEDICATION ADMINISTRATION

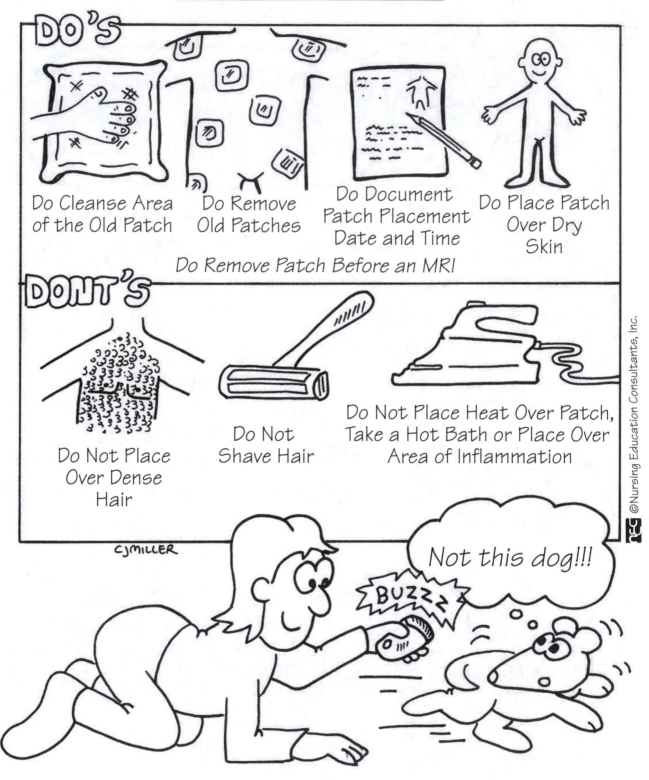

GUIDE TO DRUG OVERDOSE

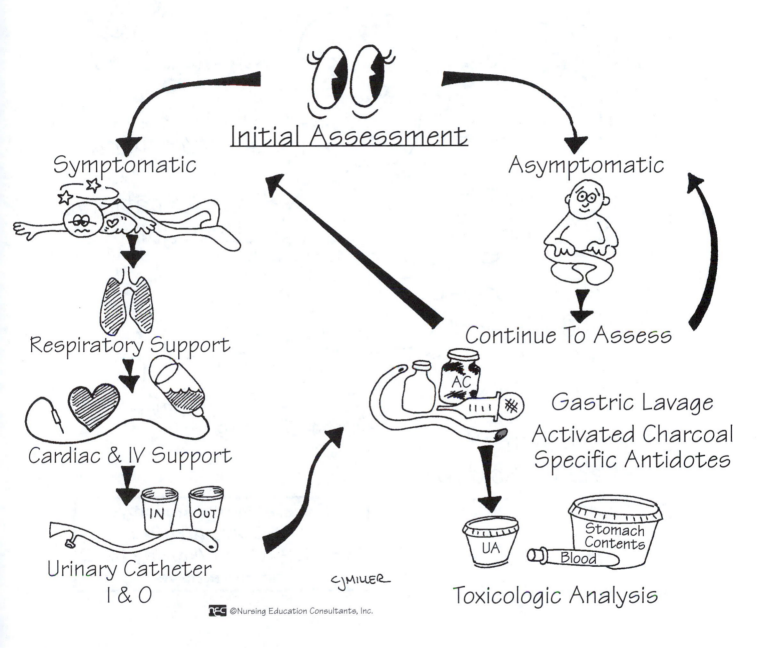

Initial Assessment

Symptomatic

Respiratory Support

Cardiac & IV Support

Urinary Catheter I & O

Asymptomatic

Continue To Assess

Gastric Lavage
Activated Charcoal
Specific Antidotes

Toxicologic Analysis

CJMILLER

SALICYLATE POISONING

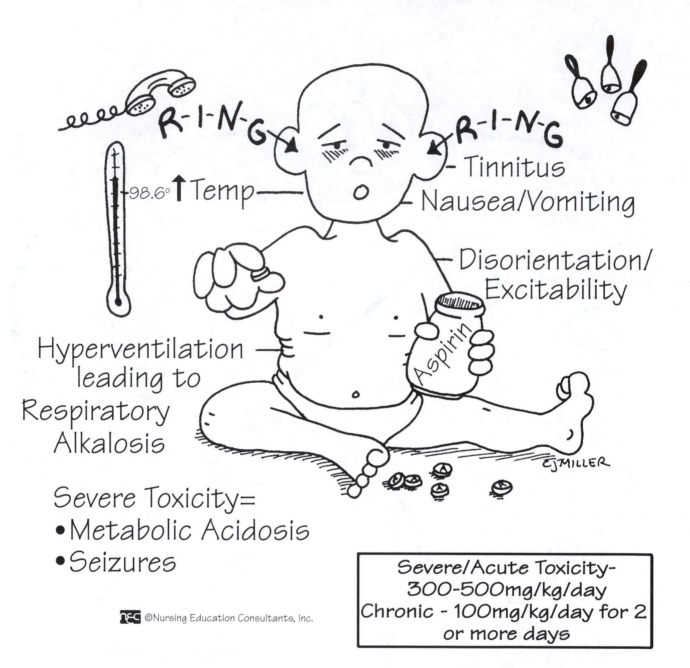

R-I-N-G   R-I-N-G

↑98.6° ↑Temp

- Tinnitus
- Nausea/Vomiting
- Disorientation/Excitability

Hyperventilation leading to Respiratory Alkalosis

Aspirin

Severe Toxicity=
- Metabolic Acidosis
- Seizures

©Nursing Education Consultants, Inc.

Severe/Acute Toxicity-
300-500mg/kg/day
Chronic - 100mg/kg/day for 2
or more days

LIDOCAINE TOXICITY

S - Slurred or Difficult Speech
- Paresthesias
- Numbness of Lips / Tongue

A - Altered Cardio-Vascular System
- Drowsiness/Dizziness/Hypotension
- Dysrhythmias - Bradycardia, Heart Block

M - Muscle Twitching
- Tremors

S - Seizures
- Confusion
- Convulsions
- Respiratory Depression

C.J.MILLER

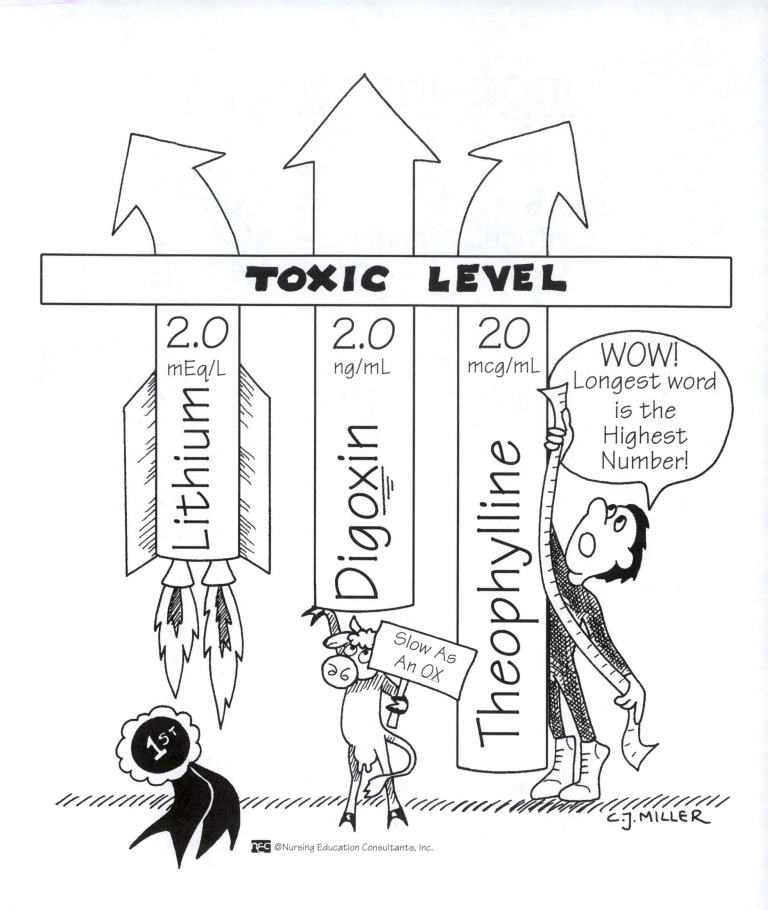

AMINOGLYCOSIDE TOXICITY

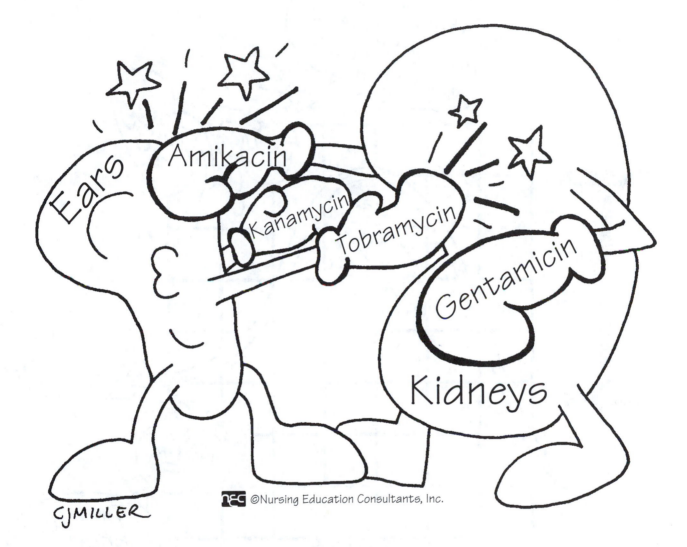

Major Toxic Effects of Aminoglycosides are Ototoxicity & Nephrotoxicity

PEAK AND TROUGH

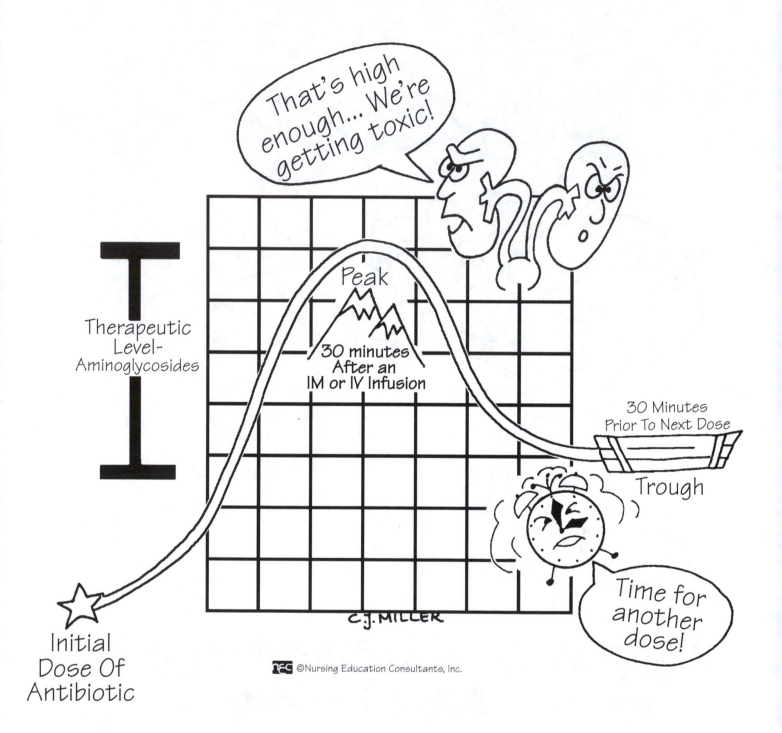

Pharmacology
NursingEd.com

SERIOUS COMPLICATIONS OF ORAL BIRTH CONTROL PILLS

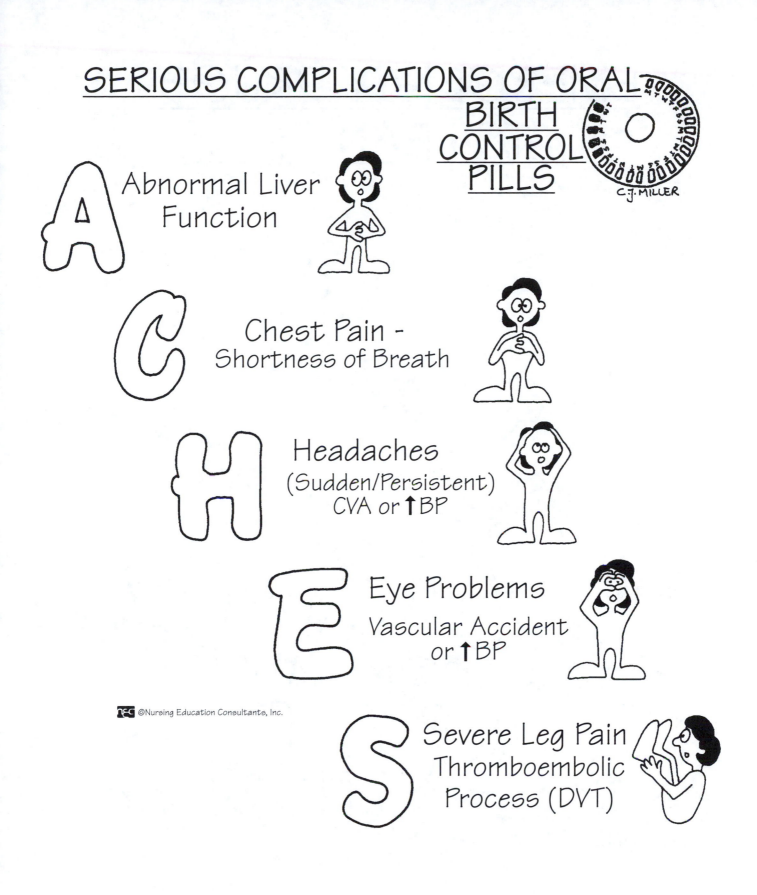

A Abnormal Liver Function

C Chest Pain - Shortness of Breath

H Headaches (Sudden/Persistent) CVA or ↑BP

E Eye Problems Vascular Accident or ↑BP

S Severe Leg Pain Thromboembolic Process (DVT)

C.J. MILLER

EMERGENCY DRUGS
TO **LEAN** ON

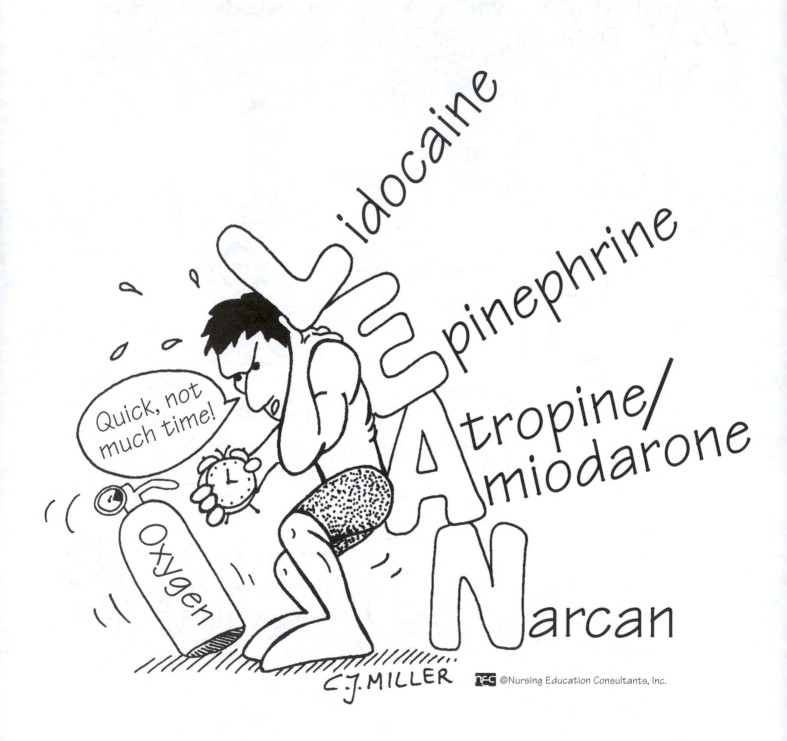

Lidocaine
Epinephrine
Atropine/Amiodarone
Narcan

Quick, not much time!

Oxygen

C.J. MILLER

©Nursing Education Consultants, Inc.

BETA BLOCKER ACTIONS

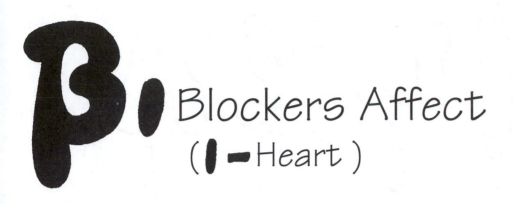 β_1 Blockers Affect
(1 - Heart)

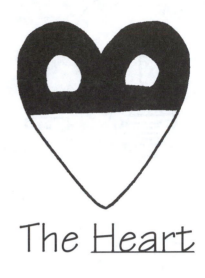

The <u>Heart</u>

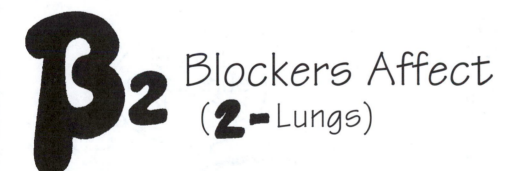 β_2 Blockers Affect
(2 - Lungs)

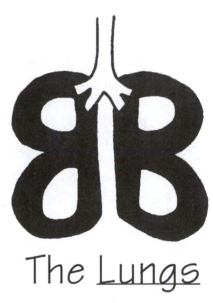

The <u>Lungs</u>

CJ MILLER

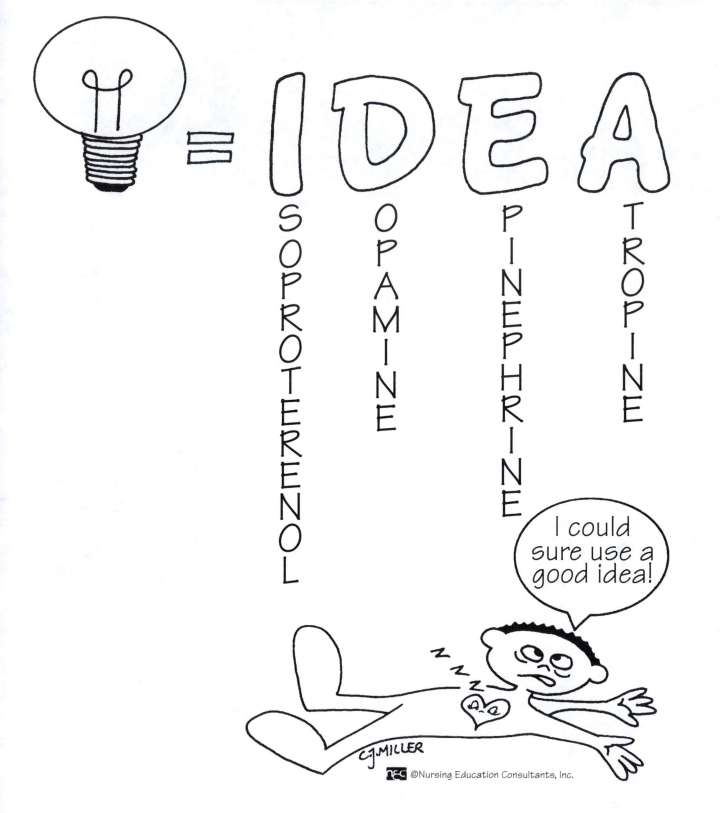

ANTI-HYPERTENSIVE DRUGS

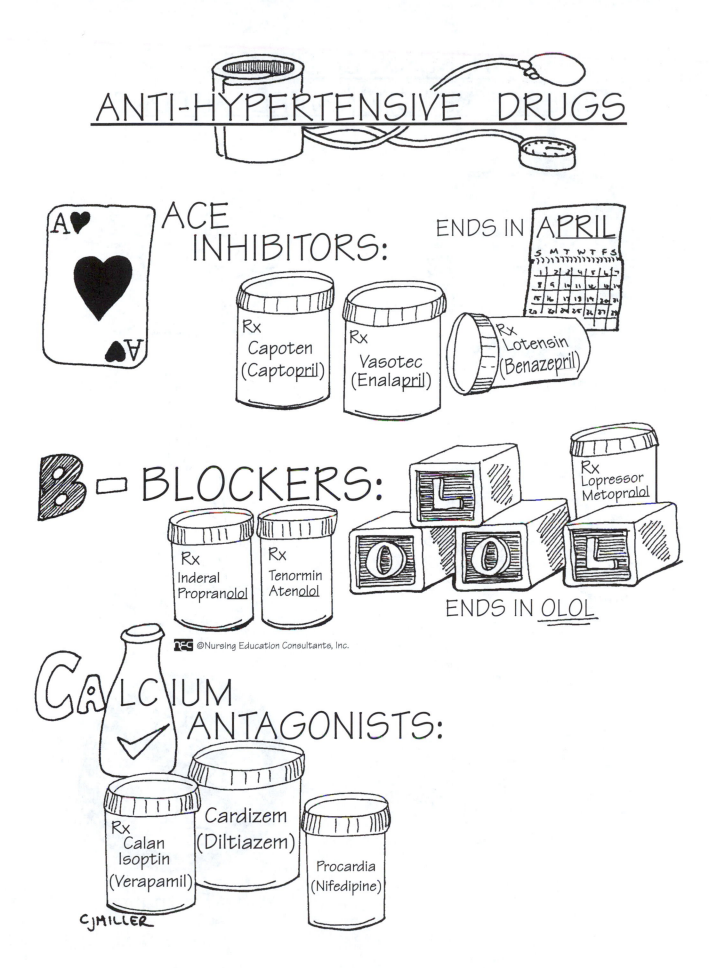

ACE INHIBITORS:

ENDS IN APRIL

Rx Capoten (Captopril)

Rx Vasotec (Enalapril)

Rx Lotensin (Benazepril)

B - BLOCKERS:

Rx Inderal Propranolol

Rx Tenormin Atenolol

LOL

ENDS IN OLOL

Rx Lopressor Metoprolol

@Nursing Education Consultants, Inc.

CALCIUM ANTAGONISTS:

Rx Calan Isoptin (Verapamil)

Cardizem (Diltiazem)

Procardia (Nifedipine)

CJMILLER

ANTI-CANCER DRUGS
ADVERSE REACTIONS/PRECAUTIONS

Bone Marrow Suppression

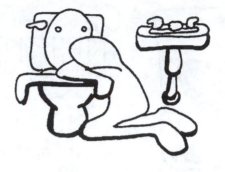

Nausea and Vomiting

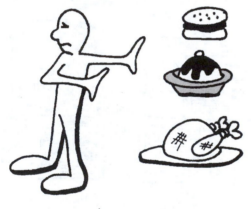

Anorexia

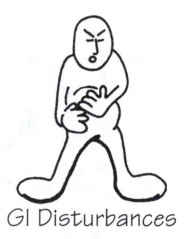

GI Disturbances

©Nursing Education Consultants, Inc.

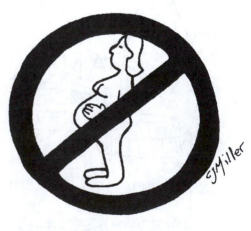

Alopecia

Avoid Pregnancy

CHOLINERGIC CRISIS

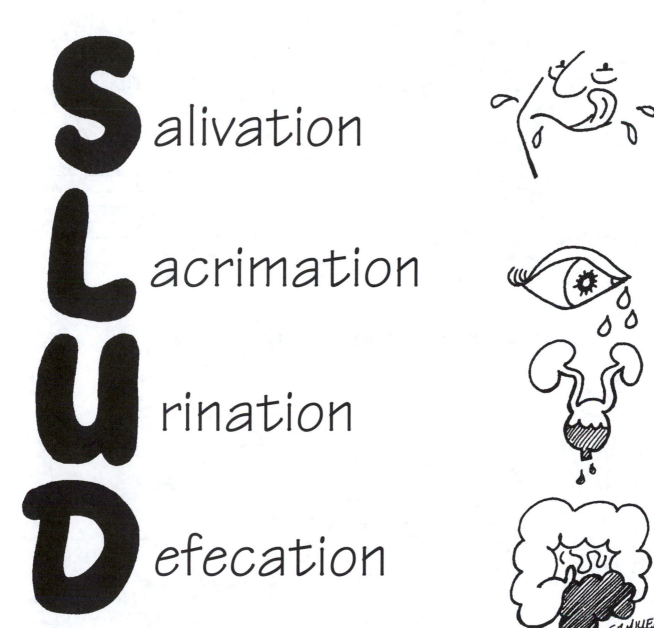

Salivation

Lacrimation

Urination

Defecation

MIXING INSULIN:

Draw Up The Clear...

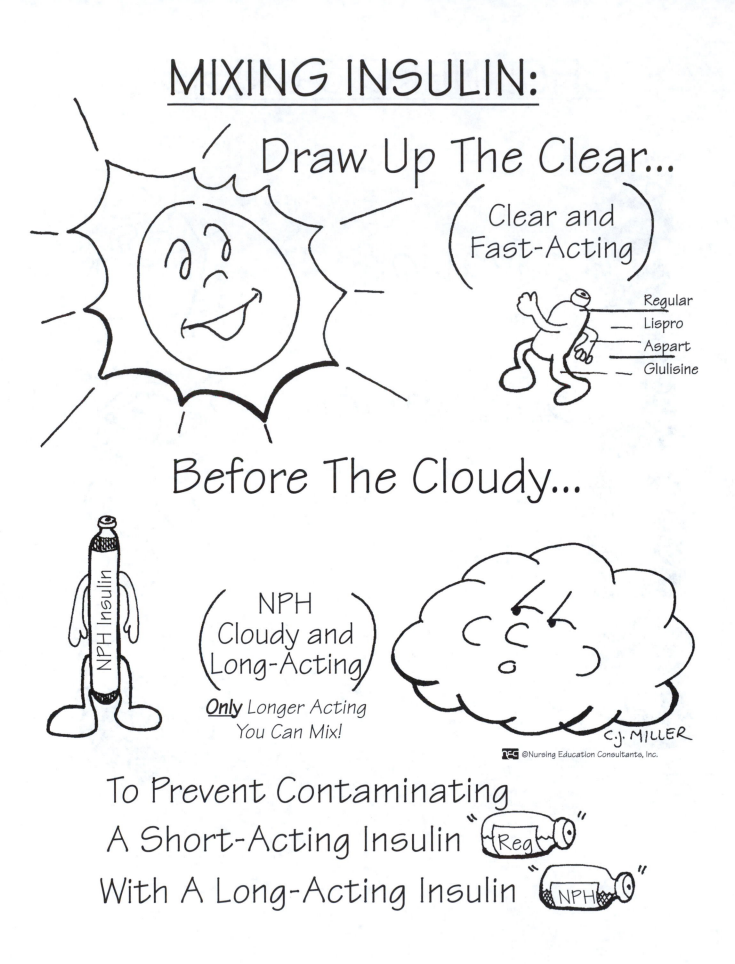

(Clear and Fast-Acting)

Regular
Lispro
Aspart
Glulisine

Before The Cloudy...

NPH Insulin

(NPH Cloudy and Long-Acting)

Only Longer Acting You Can Mix!

C.J. MILLER

©Nursing Education Consultants, Inc.

To Prevent Contaminating

A Short-Acting Insulin "Reg"

With A Long-Acting Insulin "NPH"

Pharmacology
NursingEd.com

© 2012 Nursing Education
Consultants, Inc.

HEPARIN and COUMADIN
(Corresponding Lab Tests)

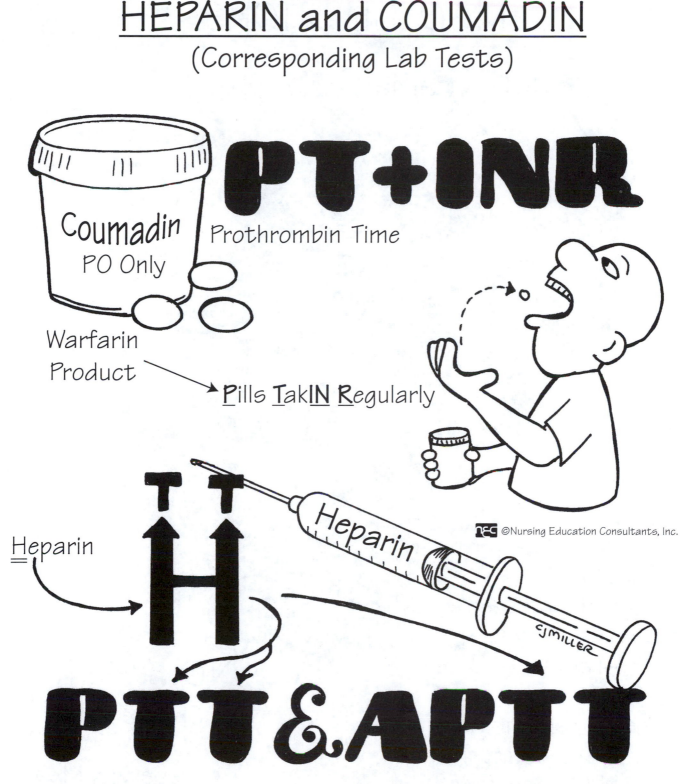

PT+INR

Prothrombin Time

Coumadin
PO Only

Warfarin
Product

Pills TakIN Regularly

Heparin

©Nursing Education Consultants, Inc.

H

PTT & APTT

Partial Thromboplastin Time & Activated Partial Thromboplastin Time

MAO INHIBITORS

Nardil **P**arnate **M**arplan

No
Popular
Meds

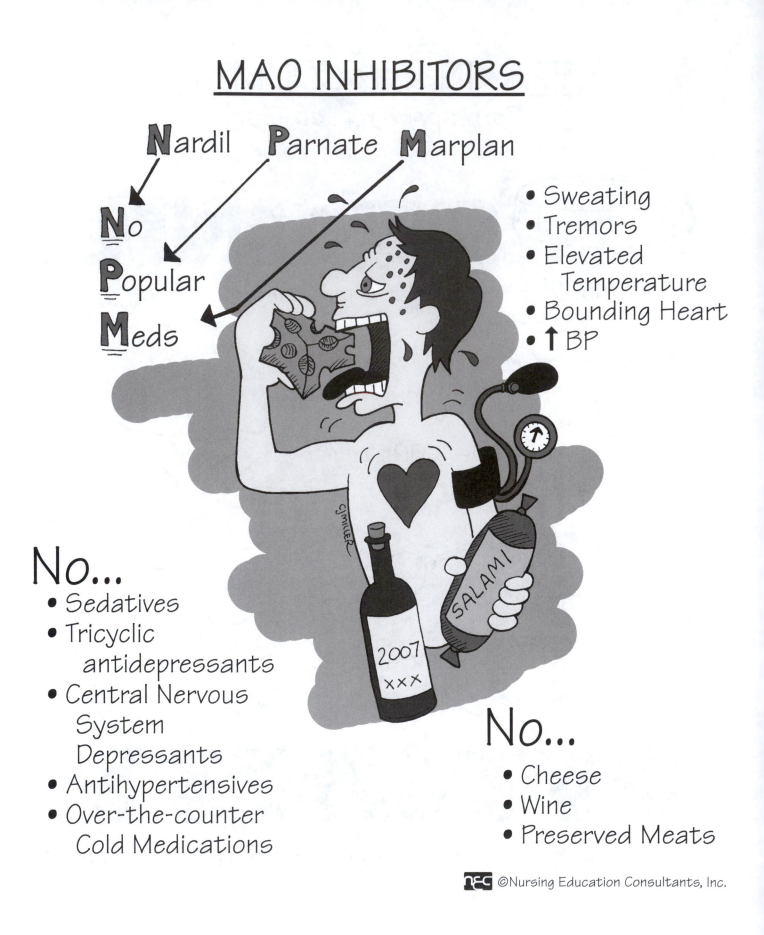

- Sweating
- Tremors
- Elevated Temperature
- Bounding Heart
- ↑ BP

No...
- Sedatives
- Tricyclic antidepressants
- Central Nervous System Depressants
- Antihypertensives
- Over-the-counter Cold Medications

No...
- Cheese
- Wine
- Preserved Meats

©Nursing Education Consultants, Inc.

ANTI-INFLAMMATORY
(Corticosteroids)

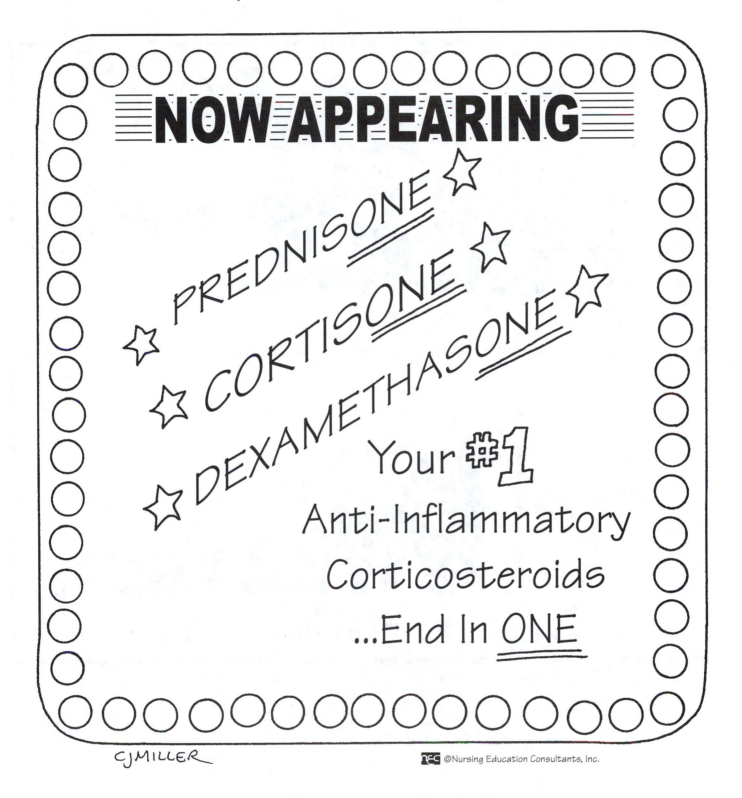

NOW APPEARING

PREDNISONE ☆

☆ CORTISONE ☆

☆ DEXAMETHASONE ☆

Your #1

Anti-Inflammatory

Corticosteroids

...End In ONE

CJMILLER

B6 - ISONIAZID and LEVODOPA

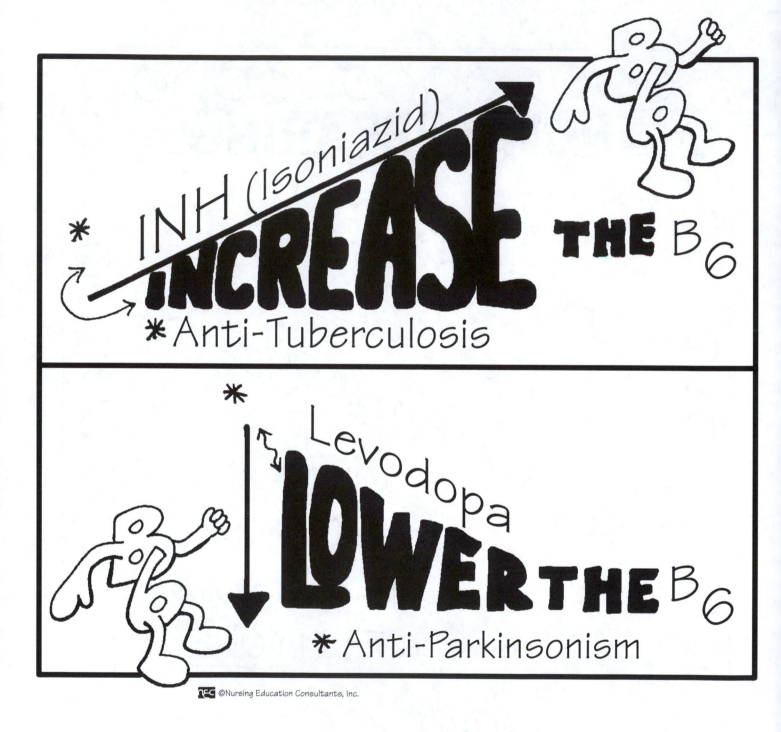

* INH (Isoniazid) INCREASE THE B6
* Anti-Tuberculosis

* Levodopa LOWER THE B6
* Anti-Parkinsonism

©Nursing Education Consultants, Inc.

INSULIN PREGNANCY REQUIREMENTS

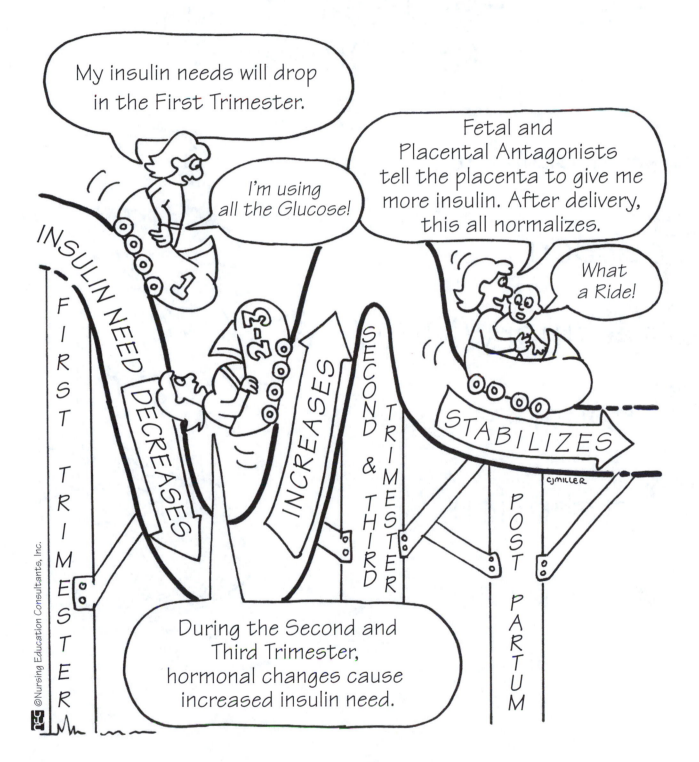

PSYCHIATRIC ASSESSMENT

Always Send Mail Through The Post Office...

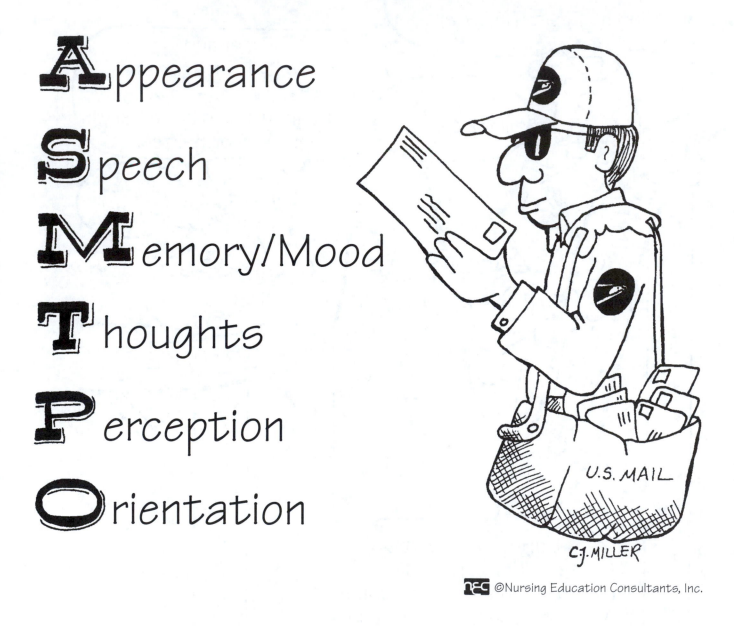

Appearance

Speech

Memory/Mood

Thoughts

Perception

Orientation

CJ.MILLER

©Nursing Education Consultants, Inc.

DEPRESSION ASSESSMENT
(SIG E CAPS)

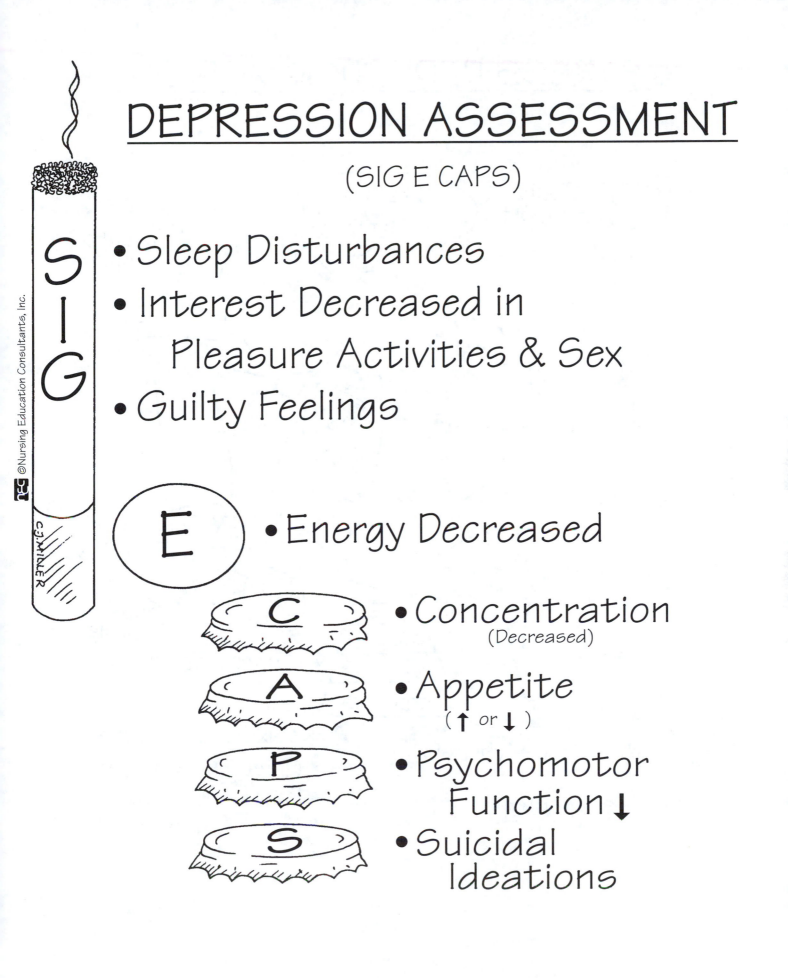

S **I** **G**
- Sleep Disturbances
- Interest Decreased in
   Pleasure Activities & Sex
- Guilty Feelings

E
- Energy Decreased

C
- Concentration
   (Decreased)

A
- Appetite
   (↑ or ↓)

P
- Psychomotor
   Function ↓

S
- Suicidal
   Ideations

C.J. MILLER

STRESS REDUCTION METHODS

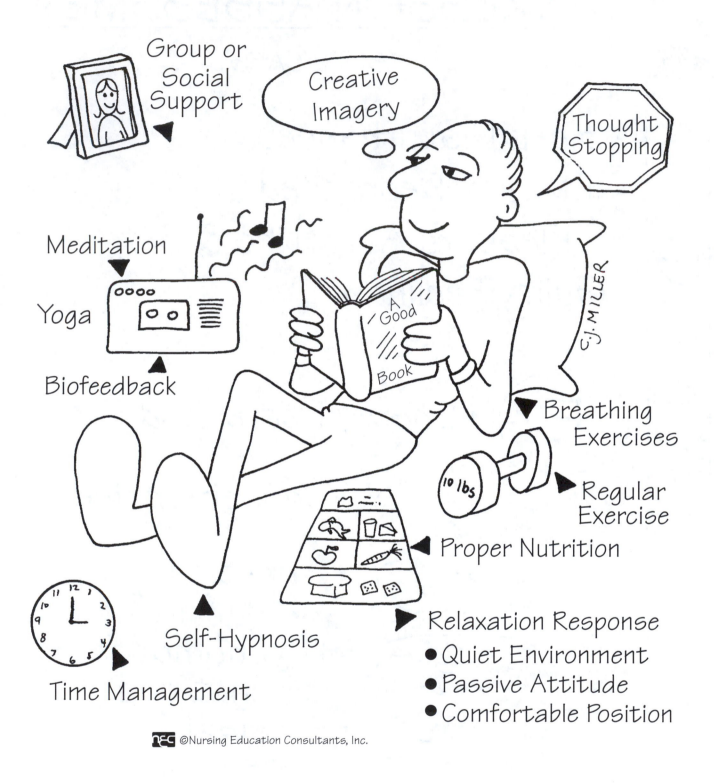

Group or Social Support

Creative Imagery

Thought Stopping

Meditation

Yoga

Biofeedback

A Good Book

Breathing Exercises

10 lbs

Regular Exercise

Proper Nutrition

Self-Hypnosis

Time Management

Relaxation Response
- Quiet Environment
- Passive Attitude
- Comfortable Position

C.J. MILLER

5 As to Alzheimer Diagnosis

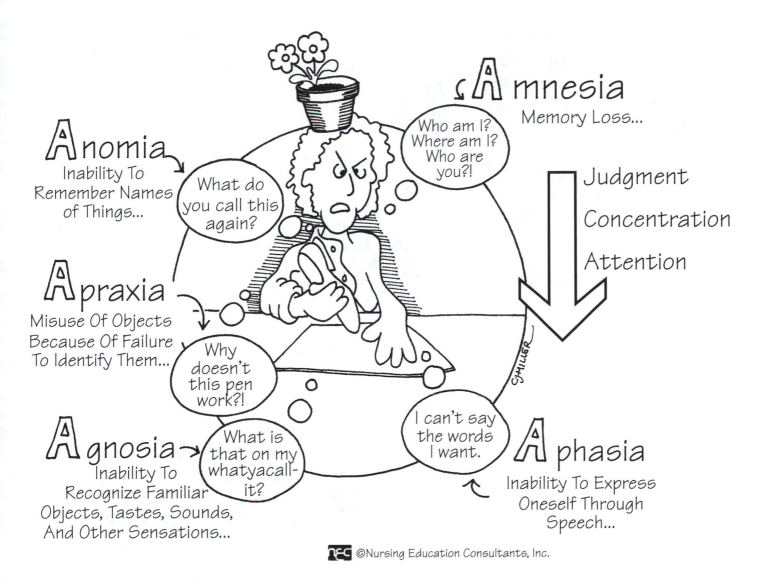

SUNDOWNING SYNDROME

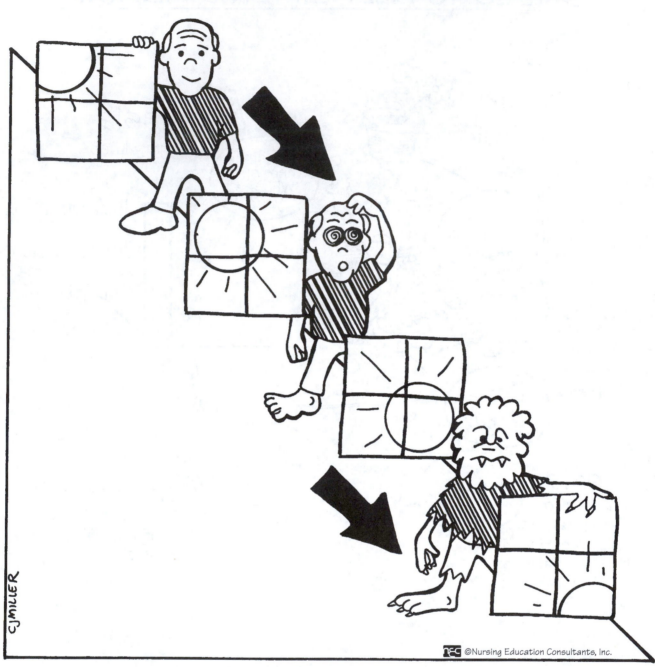

The closer to evening and "sundown," the more confused and agitated the client becomes.

Psychosocial
NursingEd.com

© 2012 Nursing Education
Consultants, Inc.

ANOREXIA NERVOSA

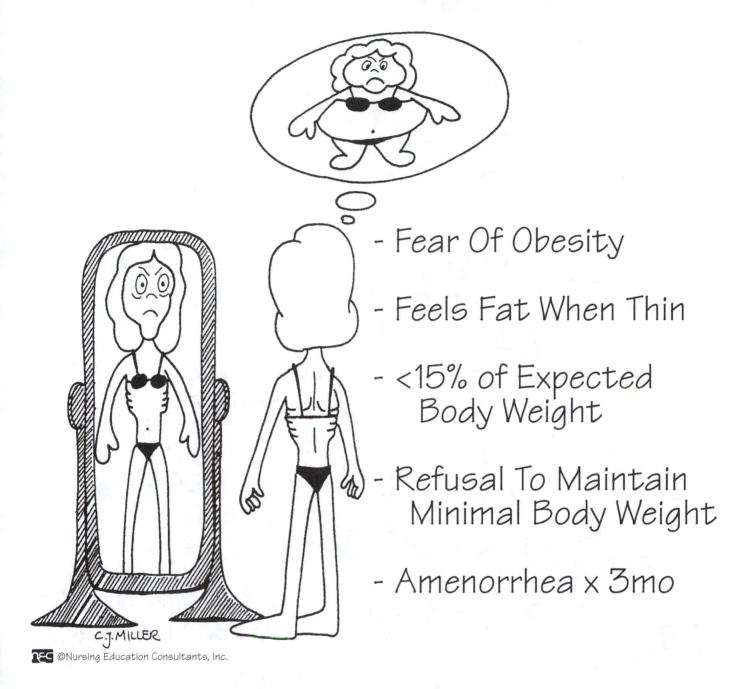

- Fear Of Obesity

- Feels Fat When Thin

- <15% of Expected Body Weight

- Refusal To Maintain Minimal Body Weight

- Amenorrhea x 3mo

C.J. MILLER

©Nursing Education Consultants, Inc.

BULIMIA

* Binge Eating
  (Usually in Solitude)
* ↑ Mood While Eating
* ↓ Mood When Stopped

©Nursing Education Consultants, Inc.

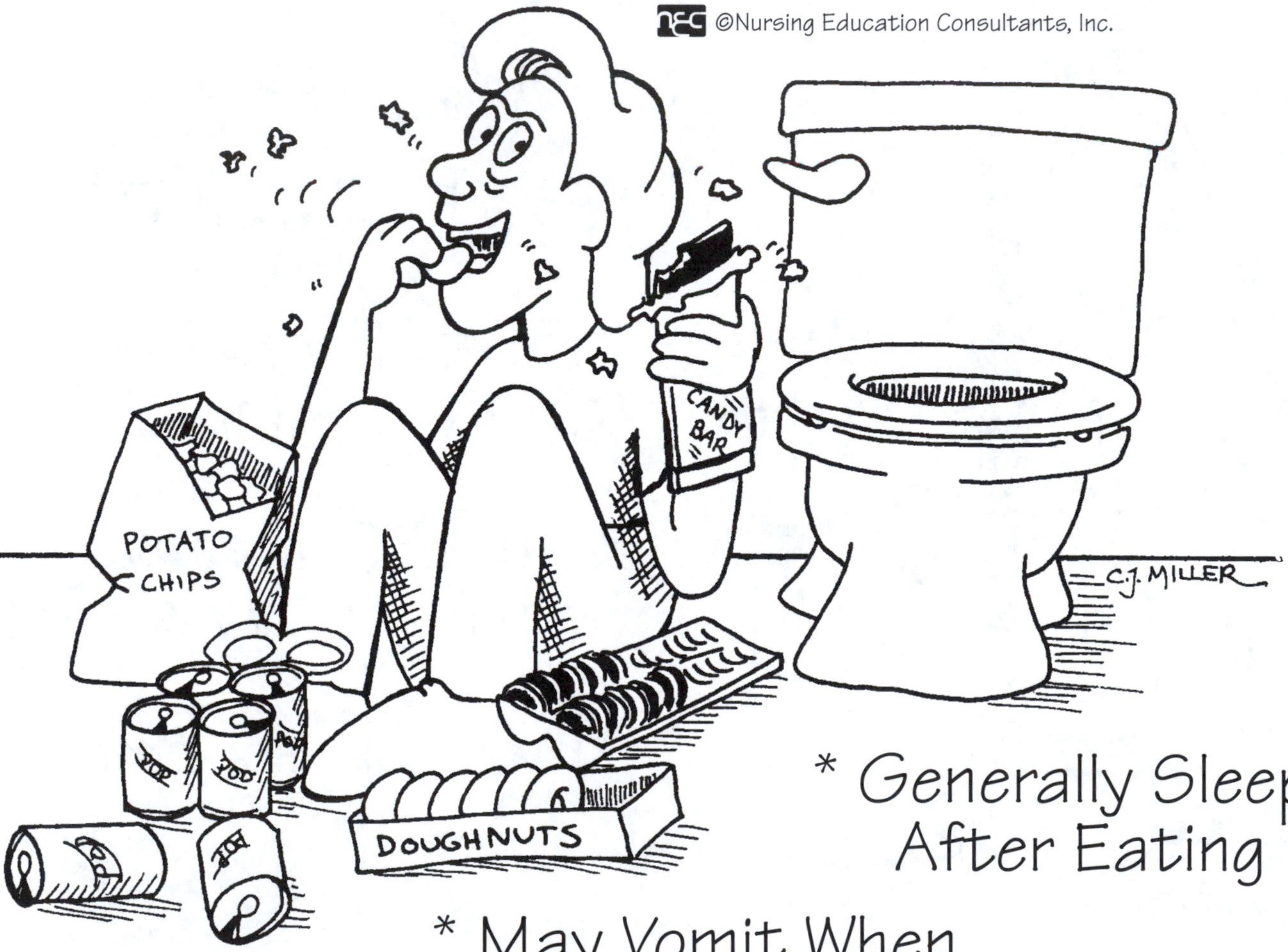

POTATO CHIPS

CANDY BAR

DOUGHNUTS

C.J. MILLER

* Generally Sleeps
  After Eating

* May Vomit When
  Binge Is Over

CHILD ABUSE

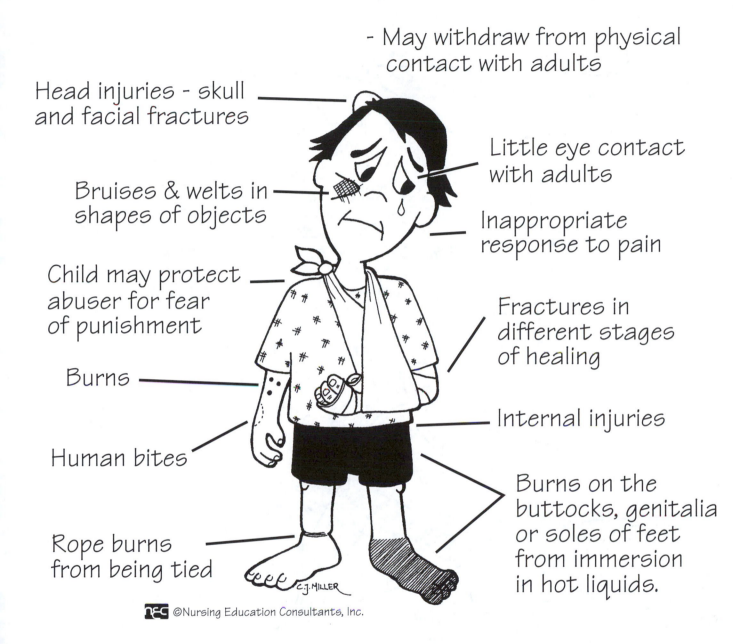

- May withdraw from physical contact with adults

Head injuries - skull and facial fractures

Little eye contact with adults

Bruises & welts in shapes of objects

Inappropriate response to pain

Child may protect abuser for fear of punishment

Fractures in different stages of healing

Burns

Internal injuries

Human bites

Burns on the buttocks, genitalia or soles of feet from immersion in hot liquids.

Rope burns from being tied

C.J. MILLER

©Nursing Education Consultants, Inc.

Psychosocial
NursingEd.com

OBSESSIVE-COMPULSIVE DISORDER

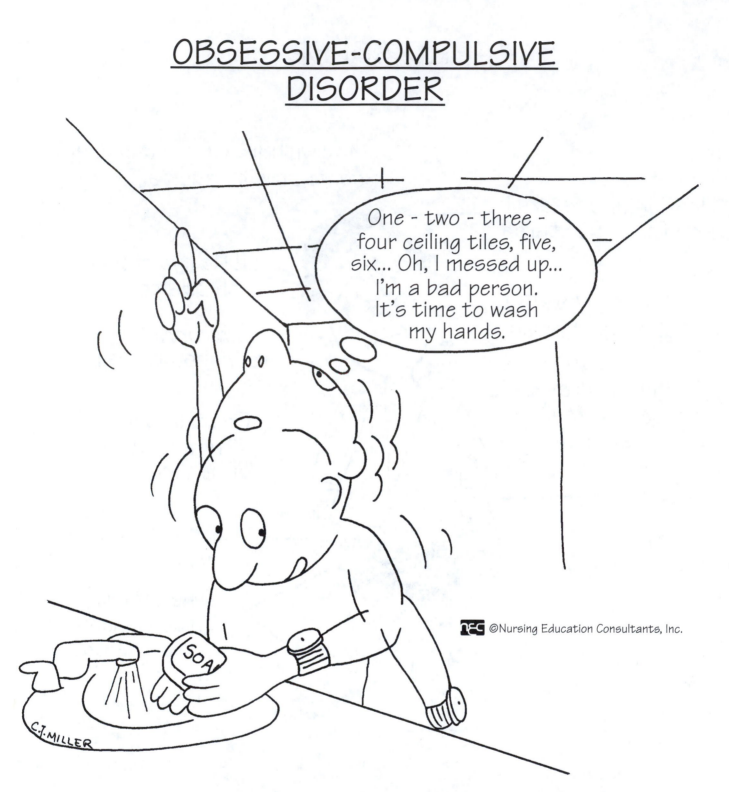

Thoughts = Obsessions = "I'm so bad; I made a mistake."
Actions = Compulsions = "I'd better wash my hands."

MANIC ATTACK - PRIMARY SYMPTOMS

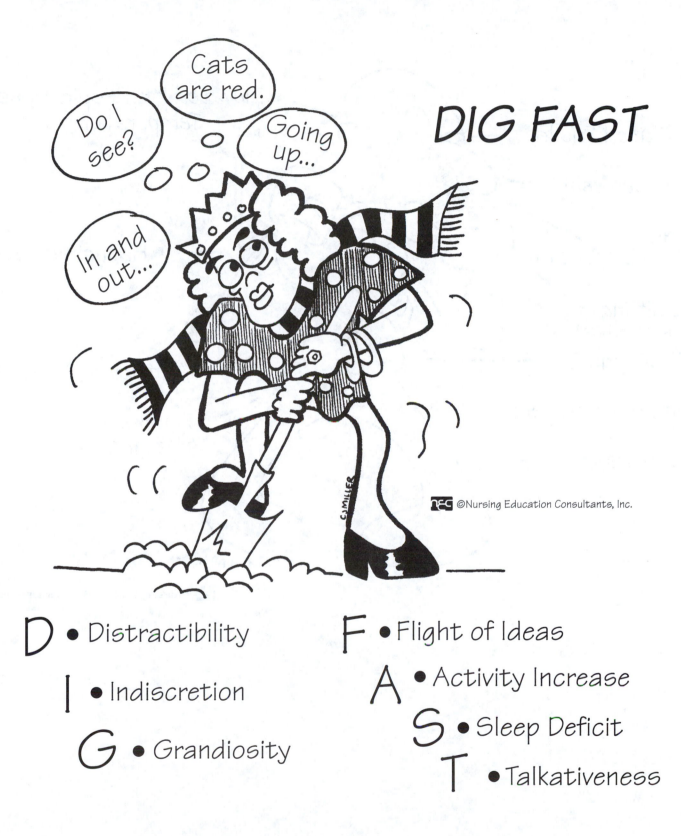

DIG FAST

D • Distractibility

I • Indiscretion

G • Grandiosity

F • Flight of Ideas

A • Activity Increase

S • Sleep Deficit

T • Talkativeness

Psychosocial
NursingEd.com

COCAINE / CRACK USERS

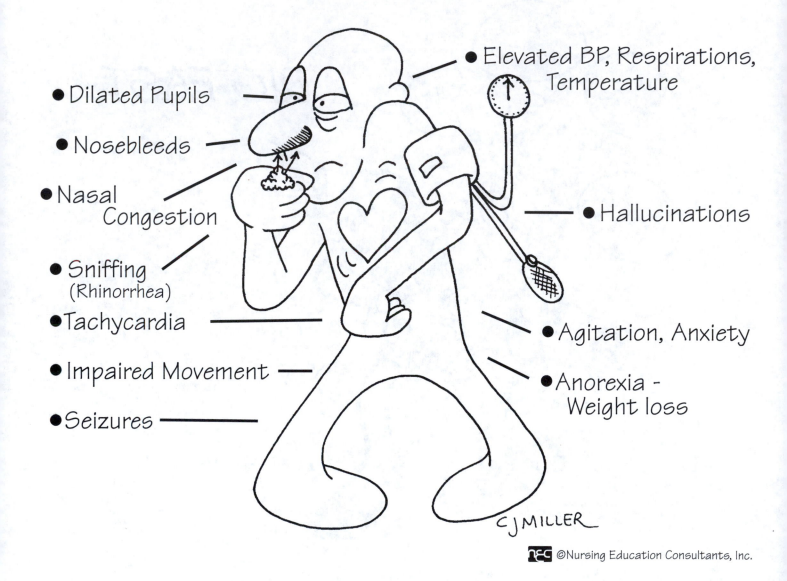

- Dilated Pupils
- Nosebleeds
- Nasal Congestion
- Sniffing (Rhinorrhea)
- Tachycardia
- Impaired Movement
- Seizures
- Elevated BP, Respirations, Temperature
- Hallucinations
- Agitation, Anxiety
- Anorexia - Weight loss

CJ MILLER

©Nursing Education Consultants, Inc.

DEMENTIA

Make Sure The Client Doesn't Have Any Problems With:

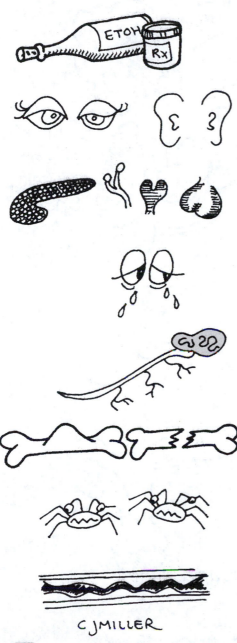

Drug/Alcohol/Depression

Eyes & Ears

Metabolic & Endocrine Disorders

Emotional Disorders

Neurologic Disorders

Tumors & Trauma

Infection/Cystitis

Arteriovascular Disease

CJMILLER

SYSTEMIC LUPUS ERYTHEMATOSUS (SLE)

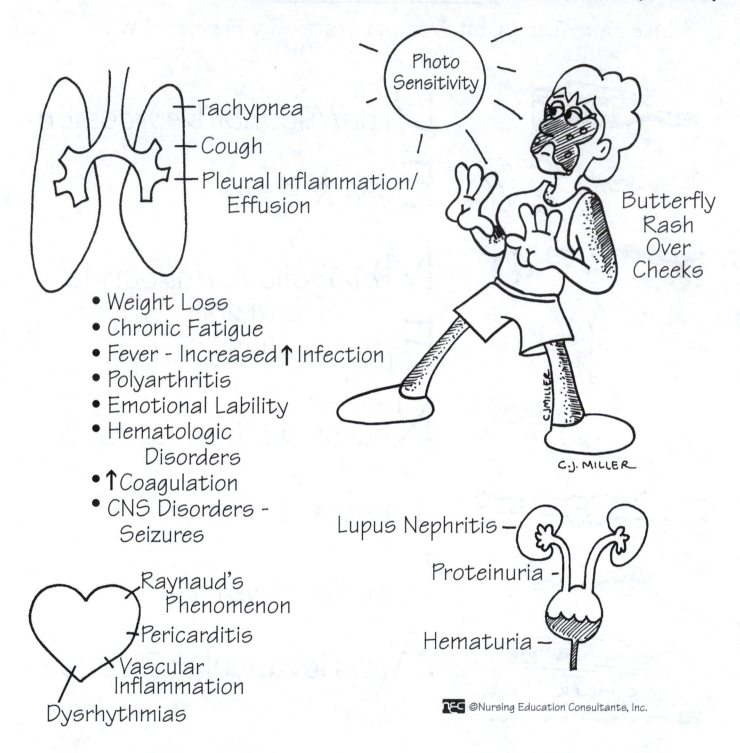

- Tachypnea
- Cough
- Pleural Inflammation/ Effusion

Photo Sensitivity

Butterfly Rash Over Cheeks

- Weight Loss
- Chronic Fatigue
- Fever - Increased ↑ Infection
- Polyarthritis
- Emotional Lability
- Hematologic Disorders
- ↑ Coagulation
- CNS Disorders - Seizures

Raynaud's Phenomenon
Pericarditis
Vascular Inflammation
Dysrhythmias

Lupus Nephritis —
Proteinuria -
Hematuria —

C.J. MILLER

ANAPHYLACTIC REACTION

Causes:
- Insect Stings (bee, wasp, ant)
- Medications and Latex
- Food Allergy
  (peanuts, eggs, shellfish)

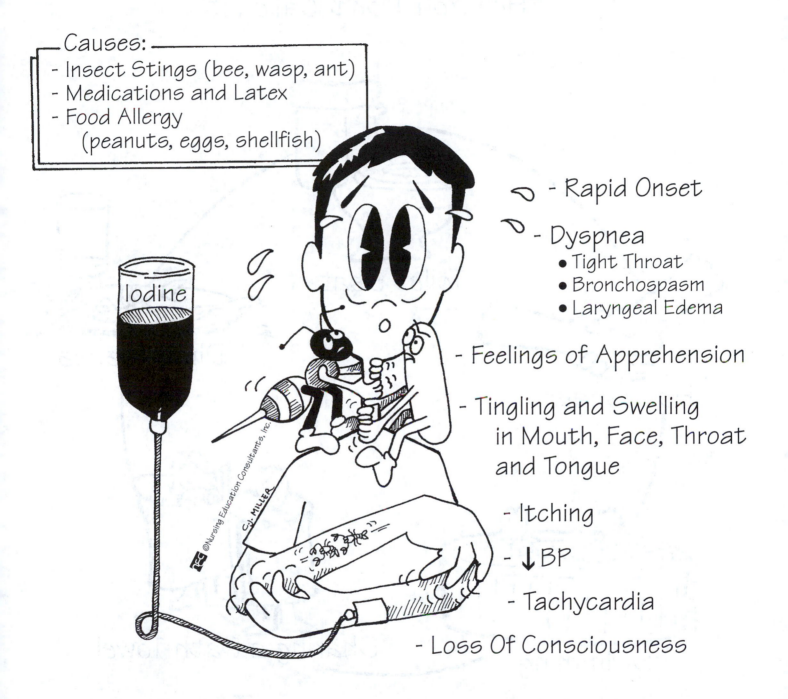

- Rapid Onset

- Dyspnea
  • Tight Throat
  • Bronchospasm
  • Laryngeal Edema

- Feelings of Apprehension

- Tingling and Swelling
  in Mouth, Face, Throat
  and Tongue

- Itching

- ↓BP

- Tachycardia

- Loss Of Consciousness

AIDS
"How You Don't Catch It"

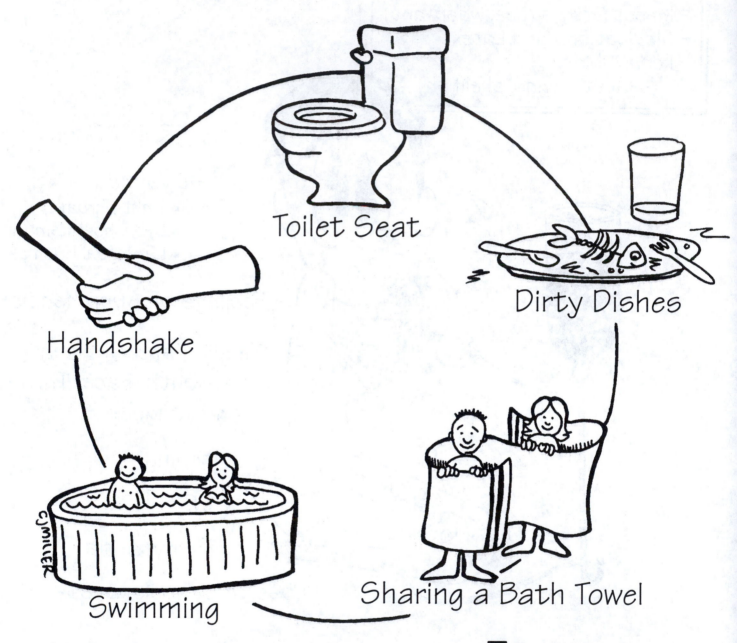

Toilet Seat

Dirty Dishes

Handshake

Sharing a Bath Towel

Swimming

©Nursing Education Consultants, Inc.

Immune
NursingEd.com

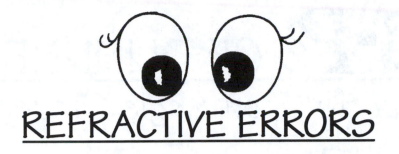

REFRACTIVE ERRORS

* <u>My</u>opia - "<u>My</u>" = <u>Near</u>sightedness
Can See Near.

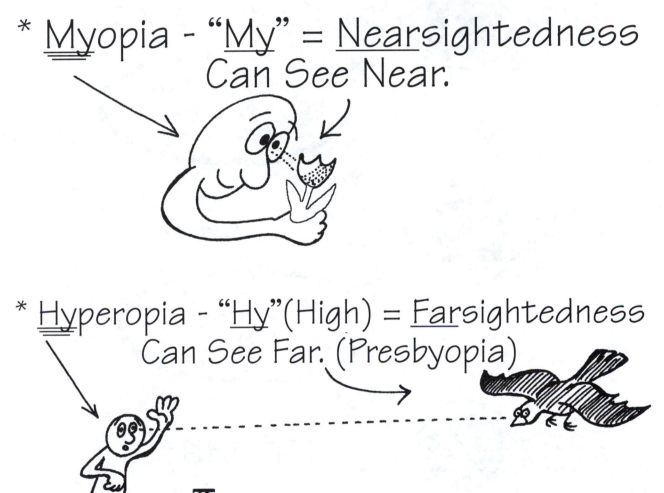

* <u>Hy</u>peropia - "<u>Hy</u>"(High) = <u>Far</u>sightedness
Can See Far. (Presbyopia)

©Nursing Education Consultants, Inc.

* Astigmatism -
↳ <u>BLURRED</u> AT ANY DISTANCE.

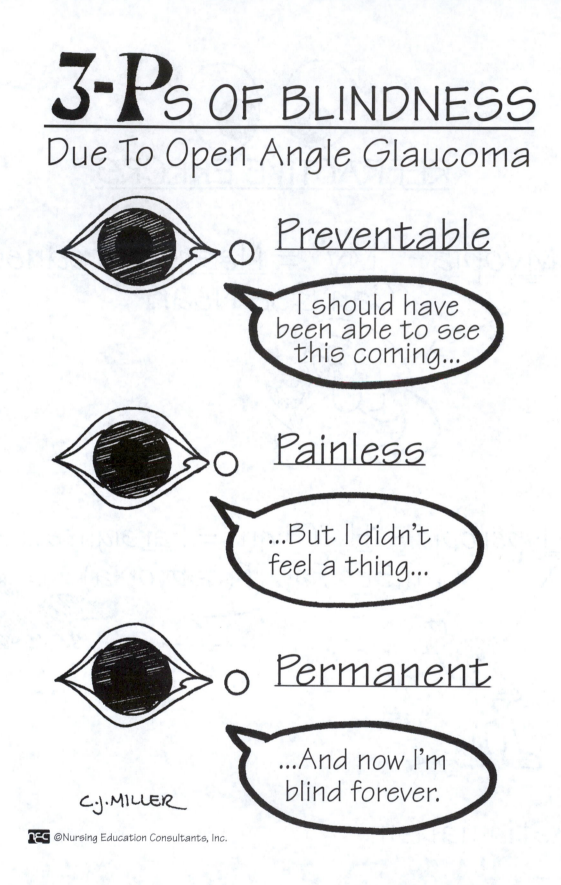

GLAUCOMA

* Increased Intraocular Pressure & Progressive Vision Loss *

Risk Factors
- Familial
- Over Age 40
- Diabetes, Hypertension
- History of Ocular Problems

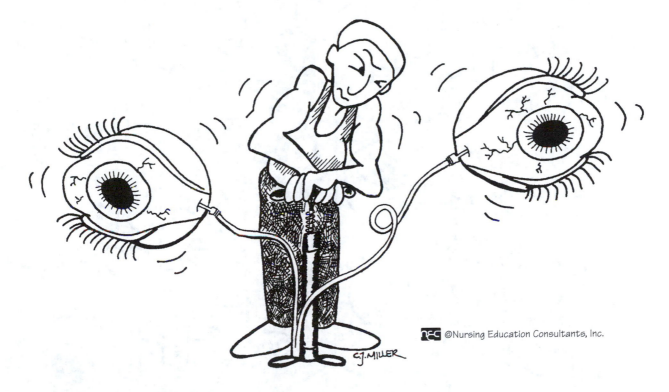

©Nursing Education Consultants, Inc.

C.J. MILLER

Primary Open-Angle Glaucoma

- Gradual Loss of Peripheral Vision (Tunnel Vision)
- Generally Painless
- Blindness if Untreated
- IOP – 22-32 mmHg
- Decreased Visual Acuity

CORNEAL TRANSPLANT SURGERY

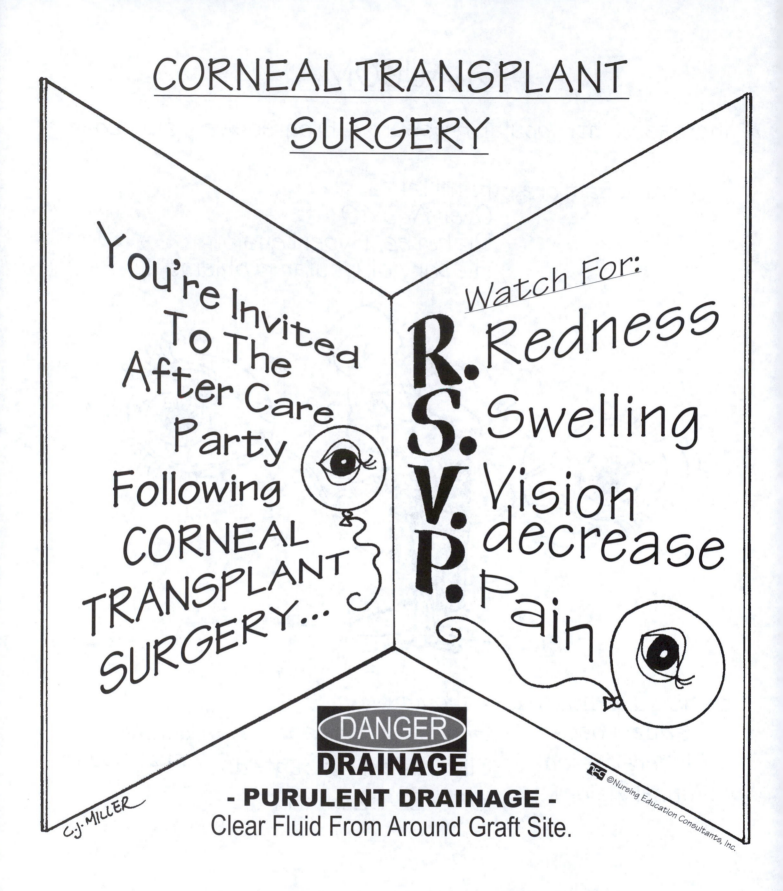

You're Invited To The After Care Party Following CORNEAL TRANSPLANT SURGERY...

Watch For:

R. Redness
S. Swelling
V. Vision decrease
P. Pain

DANGER
DRAINAGE
- PURULENT DRAINAGE -
Clear Fluid From Around Graft Site.

C.J. MILLER

©Nursing Education Consultants, Inc.

Sensory
NursingEd.com

OTITIS MEDIA

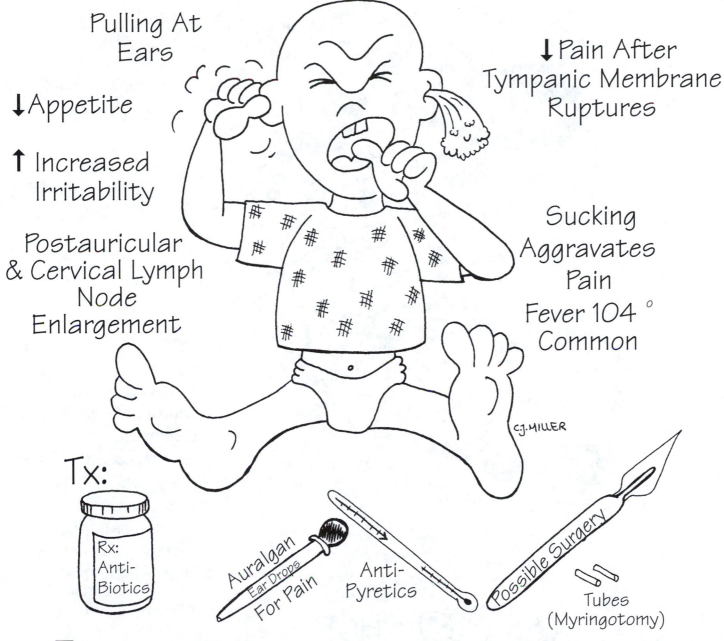

Pulling At Ears

↓Appetite

↑ Increased Irritability

Postauricular & Cervical Lymph Node Enlargement

↓Pain After Tympanic Membrane Ruptures

Sucking Aggravates Pain

Fever 104° Common

C.J. MILLER

Tx:

Rx: Anti- Biotics

Auralgan Ear Drops For Pain

Anti- Pyretics

Possible Surgery

Tubes (Myringotomy)

SICKLE CELL ANEMIA CRISIS

(Inherited Red Blood Cell Disorder)

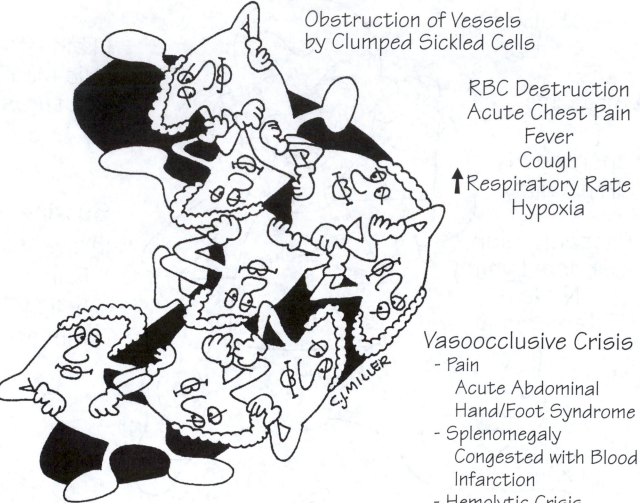

Obstruction of Vessels
by Clumped Sickled Cells

RBC Destruction
Acute Chest Pain
Fever
Cough
↑Respiratory Rate
Hypoxia

Vasoocclusive Crisis
- Pain
    Acute Abdominal
    Hand/Foot Syndrome
- Splenomegaly
    Congested with Blood
    Infarction
- Hemolytic Crisis
    Anemia, Jaundice
- Stroke (Cerebral Infarction)
- Kidney - Ischemia

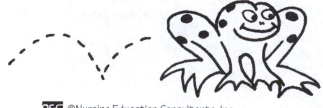

HOP -
Hydration and Electrolytes
Oxygen - Bed Rest to ↓O₂ needs
Pain Relief

HEMOPHILIA

(Inherited Blood Disorder
Factor VIII, Classic, or Type A)

- Avoid Injury

- No Cure

- Avoid Meds That
  ↑Bleeding

ASA NO NSAIDs

- Good Nutrition

- Good Dental
  Hygiene

- IV Administration
  Of Deficient
  Clotting
  Factor

Intracranial
Hemorrhage

Prolonged
Nosebleeds

Bruises Easily

Warm, Painful,
Swollen Joints
With ↓ Movement

GI Hemorrhage

COFFEE-GROUND EMESIS

COLA-COLORED URINE

TARRY STOOLS

CJMILLER

SYMPTOMS OF LEUKEMIA

A o Anemia - ↓Hgb

N o Neutropenia - Risk of infection

T o Thrombocytopenia - Bleeding

IMMATURE WHITE BLOOD CELLS

©Nursing Education Consultants, Inc.

Think ...

Leukemias = Numerous immature white blood cells like ants in an ant colony.

CJ MILLER

TYPE 2 DIABETES

Genetic Mutations = Insulin Resistance & Familial Tendency

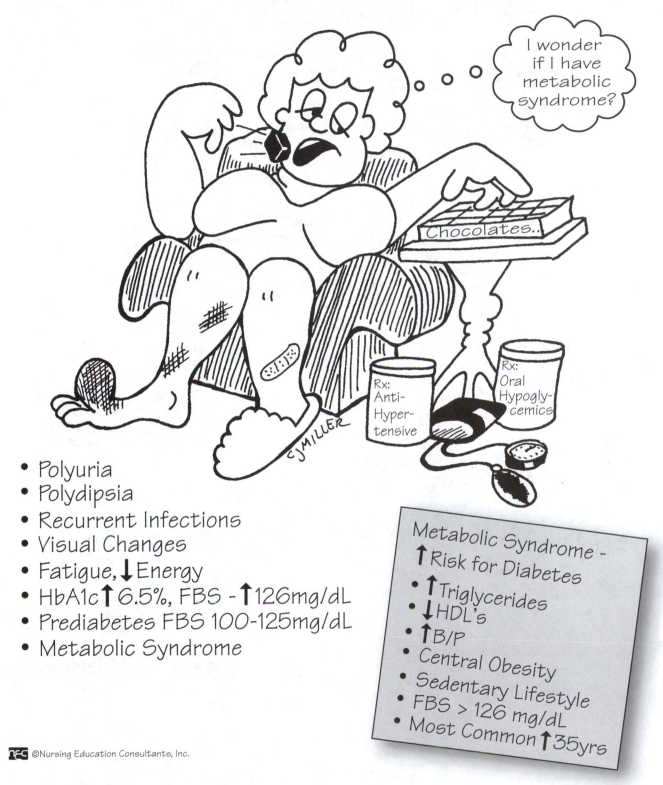

I wonder if I have metabolic syndrome?

Chocolates...

Rx: Anti-Hyper-tensive

Rx: Oral Hypogly-cemics

CJMILLER

- Polyuria
- Polydipsia
- Recurrent Infections
- Visual Changes
- Fatigue, ↓Energy
- HbA1c ↑6.5%, FBS - ↑126mg/dL
- Prediabetes FBS 100-125mg/dL
- Metabolic Syndrome

Metabolic Syndrome -
↑Risk for Diabetes
- ↑Triglycerides
- ↓HDL's
- ↑B/P
- Central Obesity
- Sedentary Lifestyle
- FBS > 126 mg/dL
- Most Common ↑35yrs

HYPOGLYCEMIA

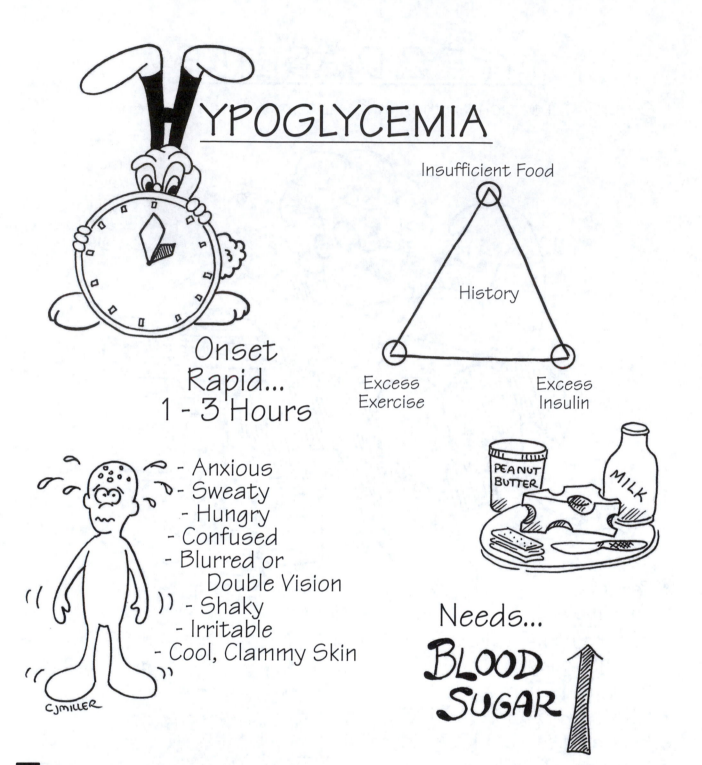

Onset
Rapid...
1 - 3 Hours

Insufficient Food

History

Excess
Exercise

Excess
Insulin

- Anxious
- Sweaty
- Hungry
- Confused
- Blurred or
  Double Vision
- Shaky
- Irritable
- Cool, Clammy Skin

PEANUT BUTTER

MILK

Needs...

BLOOD SUGAR ↑

Increased > 70mg/dL

CJMILLER

DIABETIC KETOACIDOSIS

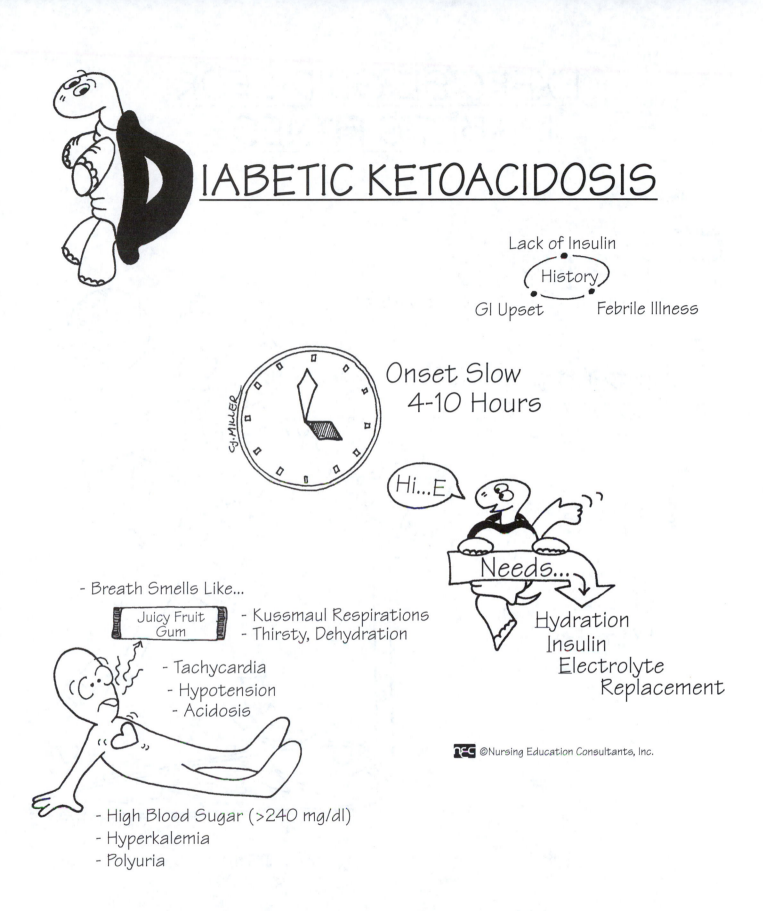

Lack of Insulin

History

GI Upset   Febrile Illness

Onset Slow
4-10 Hours

Hi...E

Needs...

Hydration
Insulin
Electrolyte
Replacement

- Breath Smells Like...

Juicy Fruit Gum

- Kussmaul Respirations
- Thirsty, Dehydration

- Tachycardia
- Hypotension
- Acidosis

- High Blood Sugar (>240 mg/dl)
- Hyperkalemia
- Polyuria

©Nursing Education Consultants, Inc.

EXERCISE GUIDE FOR DIABETIC FITNESS

F Frequency
Regular (3x to 4x Per Week)

I Intensity
60-80% Of Maximal
Heart Rate

T Time
Aerobic Activity
20-30 Min.
With 5-10 Min.
Warm Up

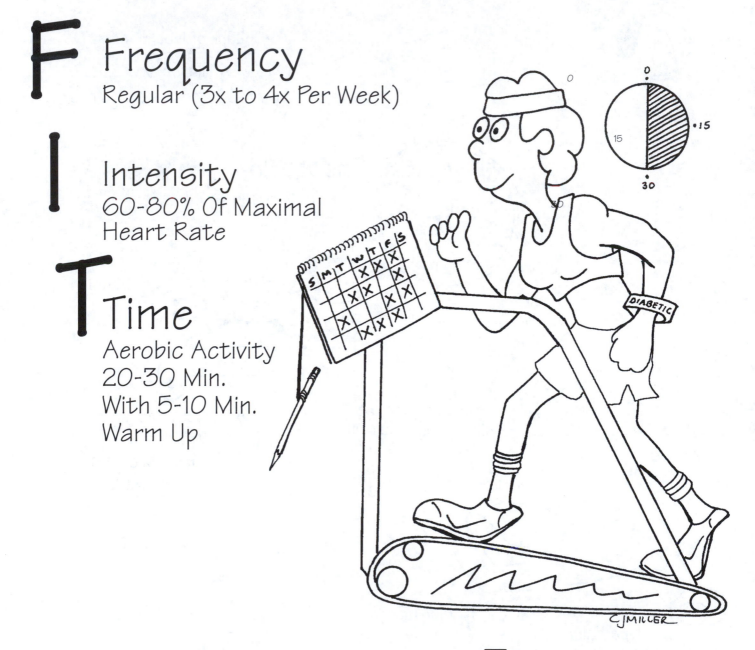

CJMILLER

©Nursing Education Consultants, Inc.

Endocrine
NursingEd.com

HYPERPITUITARY-ACROMEGALY

* Diagnosis - ↑ Plasma Insulin-like Growth Factor (IGF-1)
CT Scan, MRI
Oral Glucose Tolerance Test (OGTT) -
(Glucose Level Does Not Drop)

* Complications - Cardiac/Respiratory Problems
Diabetes

* Clinical Manifestations -

Enlarged Pituitary
- Headaches
- Visual Problems

Facial Changes
- Slanting Forehead
- Coarse Facial Features
- Protruding Jaw

Hypertrophy of Soft Tissue
Menstrual Changes
Enlargement Of Small Bones
in Hands and Feet

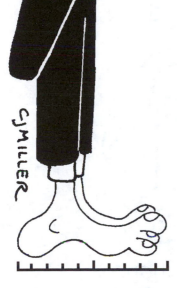

©Nursing Education Consultants, Inc.

SYMPTOMS OF HYPOXIA

Early

R - Restlessness
A - Anxiety
T - Tachycardia/Tachypnea

is Late to

B - Bradycardia
E - Extreme Restlessness
D - Dyspnea (Severe)

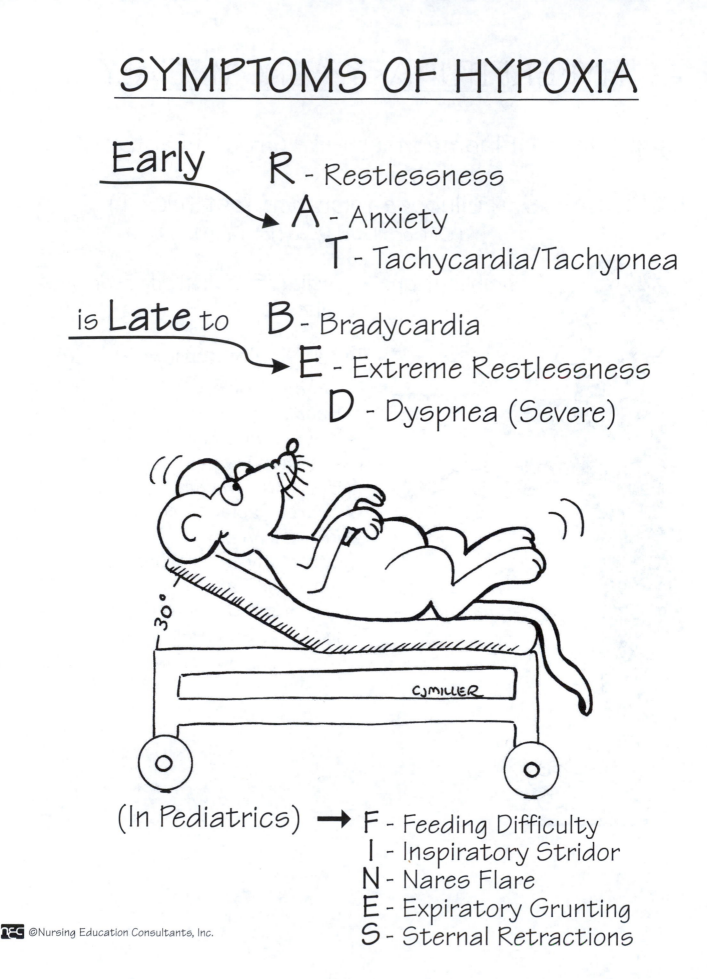

(In Pediatrics) →

F - Feeding Difficulty
I - Inspiratory Stridor
N - Nares Flare
E - Expiratory Grunting
S - Sternal Retractions

30°

CJMILLER

Respiratory
NursingEd.com

RESPIRATORY PATTERNS

Kussmaul -

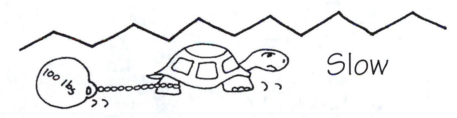

Fruity Acetone Breath

Increase in Rate and Depth

Tachypnea -

Fast

Bradypnea -

100 lb

Slow

Biots -

3-4 Irregular Breaths Then a Period Apnea

Cheyne-Stokes -

STOP   STOP   STOP

CJMILLER

Near Death Breathing Pattern

MANAGEMENT OF ASTHMA

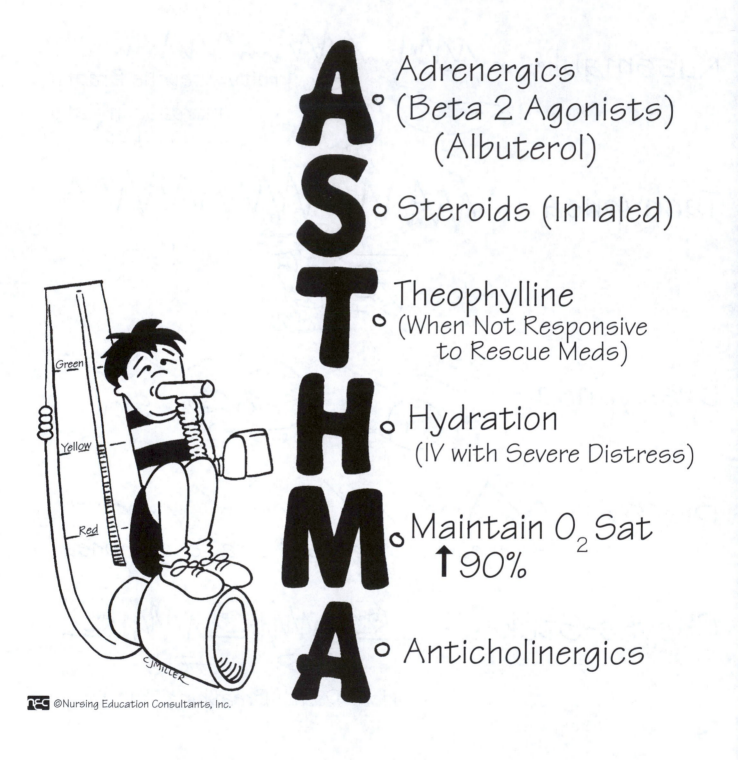

A ° Adrenergics (Beta 2 Agonists) (Albuterol)

S ° Steroids (Inhaled)

T ° Theophylline (When Not Responsive to Rescue Meds)

H ° Hydration (IV with Severe Distress)

M ° Maintain O_2 Sat ↑90%

A ° Anticholinergics

Green
Yellow
Red

CJMILLER

PNEUMO THORAX O_2

Air in the pleural cavity, resulting in lung collapse...

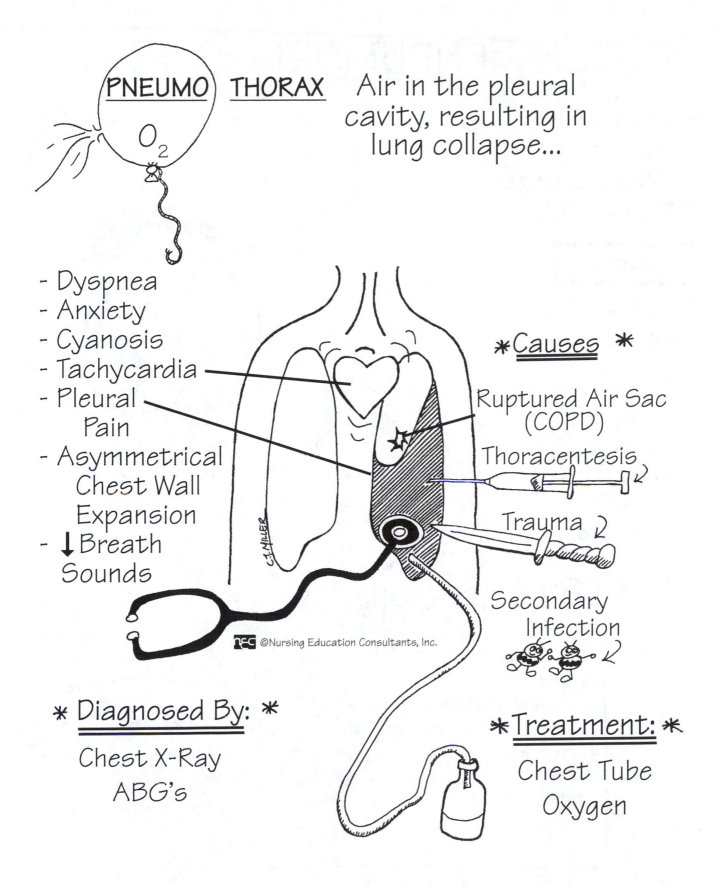

- Dyspnea
- Anxiety
- Cyanosis
- Tachycardia
- Pleural Pain
- Asymmetrical Chest Wall Expansion
- ↓ Breath Sounds

*Causes *

Ruptured Air Sac (COPD)

Thoracentesis

Trauma

Secondary Infection

* Diagnosed By: *

Chest X-Ray
ABG's

*Treatment: *

Chest Tube
Oxygen

©Nursing Education Consultants, Inc.

PNEUMONIA

- Obstruction of Bronchioles
- ↓ Gas Exchange
- ↑ Exudate

Symptoms...

- Cough
- Fever
- Chills
- Tachycardia
- Tachypnea
- Dyspnea
- Pleural Pain
- Malaise
- Respiratory Distress
- ↓ Breath Sounds

"I should wear a mask if I am within three feet of the patient."

Droplet Precautions

Cough Cough

102°F

Sputum Specimen

Drs Orders For Diagnosis
- Sputum Culture
- Chest X-Ray
- ABG's
DR CJ MILLER

- Productive Cough: Yellow, Bloodstreaked, Rusty Sputum = Infection
- Opportunistic: Pneumocystis jiroveci pneumonia (PCP) Mycobacterium avium complex (MAC)

nec ©Nursing Education Consultants, Inc.

ACUTE RESPIRATORY DISTRESS SYNDROME
(A R D S)

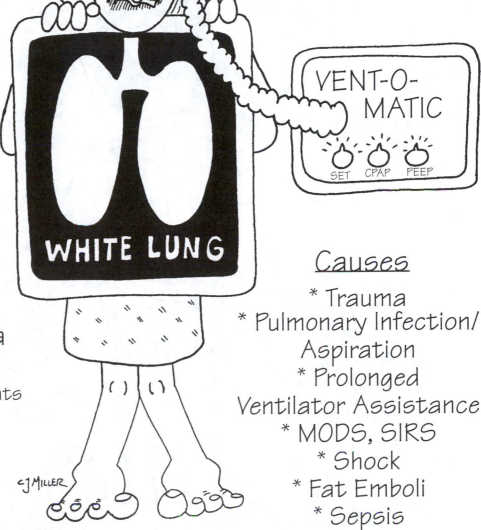

My heart is racing and I can't catch my breath

Signs & Symptoms

Tachypnea
Dyspnea
Retractions
Hypoxia
Tachycardia
↓ Pulmonary Compliance

VENT-O-MATIC

SET   CPAP   PEEP

ABGs

↓ Po_2 ↑ Dyspnea
(Refractory Hypoxia -
no improvement in O_2 sats
with ↑ FiO_2)

Causes

* Trauma
* Pulmonary Infection/ Aspiration
* Prolonged Ventilator Assistance
* MODS, SIRS
* Shock
* Fat Emboli
* Sepsis

CJ MILLER

©Nursing Education Consultants, Inc.

CYSTIC FIBROSIS (CF)

* Treatment *

- Diet - ↑ Calories & Protein
- Airway Clearance of Thick Mucus
  • Chest Physiotherapy (CPT)
  • Aerosol Bronchodilators
  • Mucolytics
- Monitor Blood Glucose
- Aerobic Exercise

- Meds
  • Antibiotics for Infection
  • Water Soluble Form of
    Vitamins A, D, E, & K
  • Pancreatic
    Enzymes

* Symptoms *

- Progressive Chronic
  Lung Disease
  • Chronic Dry Cough
  • Recurrent URI's
    (↑ Thick Sputum)
  • Chronic Hypoxia

- CF Related Diabetes (CFRD)
- Abdominal
  Distention
  - Fatigue
  - ↓ Absorption of
    Digestive Enzymes
    & Vitamins
  - Growth
    Retardation

- Rectal Prolapse
- Fatty, Stinky Stools
  (Steatorrhea)
- Meconium Ileus
  in Newborn

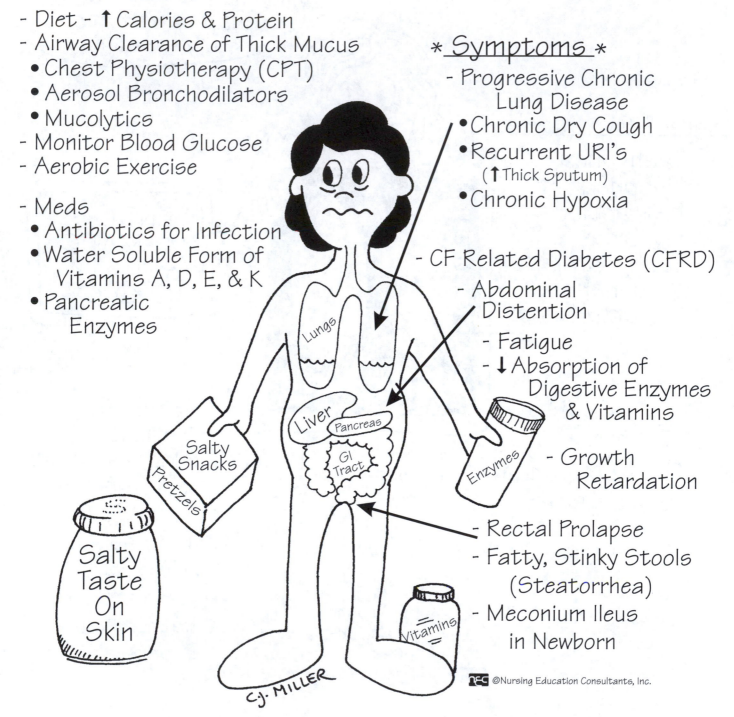

C.J. MILLER

GUIDELINES FOR PPDs

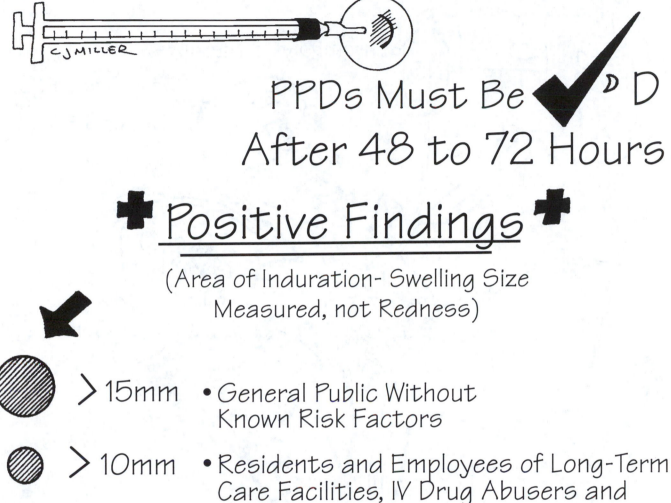

PPDs Must Be ✔ᴰ D
After 48 to 72 Hours

✚ Positive Findings ✚

(Area of Induration- Swelling Size
Measured, not Redness)

> 15mm
- General Public Without Known Risk Factors

> 10mm
- Residents and Employees of Long-Term Care Facilities, IV Drug Abusers and Recent Immigrants (< 5yrs)

> 5mm
- HIV +, Recent Contact With Active TB, Immunocompromised

PULMONARY EMBOLUS

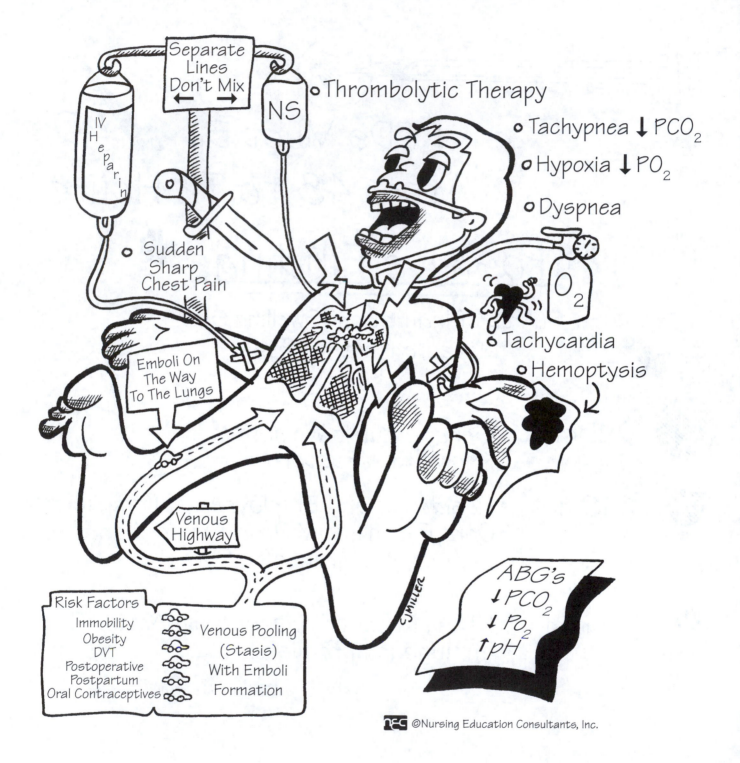

Separate Lines Don't Mix

IV Heparin

NS

Thrombolytic Therapy

Tachypnea ↓ PCO_2

Hypoxia ↓ PO_2

Dyspnea

O_2

Tachycardia

Hemoptysis

Sudden Sharp Chest Pain

Emboli On The Way To The Lungs

Venous Highway

ABG's
↓ PCO_2
↓ PO_2
↑ pH

Risk Factors

Immobility
Obesity
DVT
Postoperative
Postpartum
Oral Contraceptives

Venous Pooling (Stasis) With Emboli Formation

CJMILLER

EPIGLOTTITIS

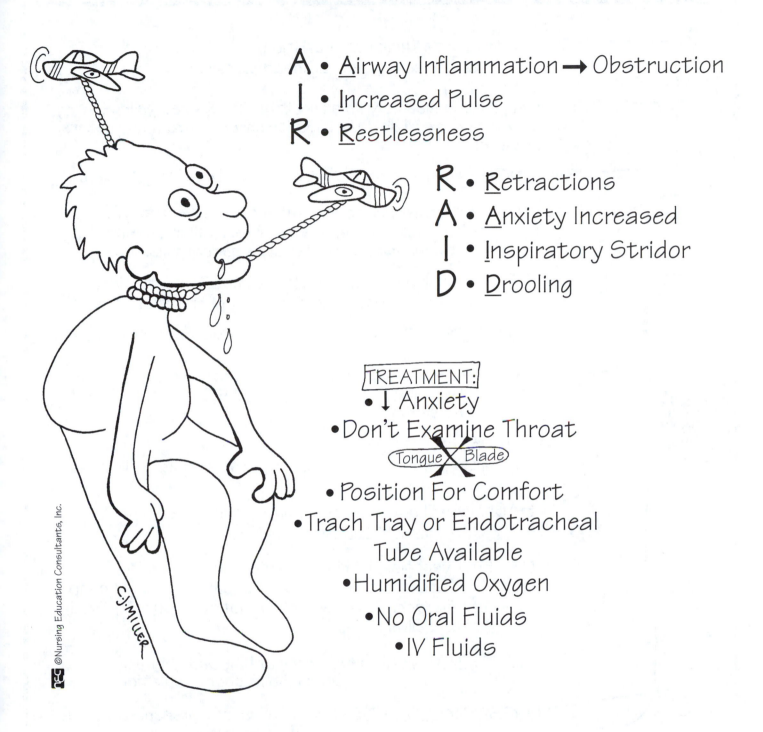

A • <u>A</u>irway Inflammation → Obstruction
I • <u>I</u>ncreased Pulse
R • <u>R</u>estlessness

R • <u>R</u>etractions
A • <u>A</u>nxiety Increased
I • <u>I</u>nspiratory Stridor
D • <u>D</u>rooling

TREATMENT:
• ↓ Anxiety
• Don't Examine Throat
  (Tongue X Blade)
• Position For Comfort
• Trach Tray or Endotracheal
  Tube Available
• Humidified Oxygen
• No Oral Fluids
• IV Fluids

CJ·MILLER

HEAD TO TOE CARDIAC CLUES

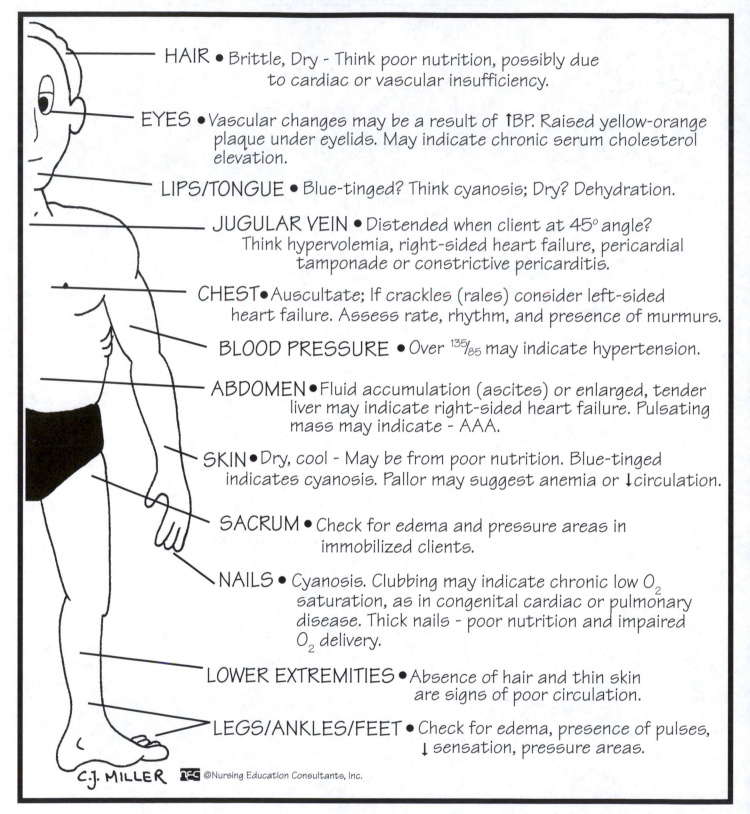

HAIR • Brittle, Dry - Think poor nutrition, possibly due to cardiac or vascular insufficiency.

EYES • Vascular changes may be a result of ↑BP. Raised yellow-orange plaque under eyelids. May indicate chronic serum cholesterol elevation.

LIPS/TONGUE • Blue-tinged? Think cyanosis; Dry? Dehydration.

JUGULAR VEIN • Distended when client at 45° angle? Think hypervolemia, right-sided heart failure, pericardial tamponade or constrictive pericarditis.

CHEST • Auscultate; If crackles (rales) consider left-sided heart failure. Assess rate, rhythm, and presence of murmurs.

BLOOD PRESSURE • Over $^{135}/_{85}$ may indicate hypertension.

ABDOMEN • Fluid accumulation (ascites) or enlarged, tender liver may indicate right-sided heart failure. Pulsating mass may indicate - AAA.

SKIN • Dry, cool - May be from poor nutrition. Blue-tinged indicates cyanosis. Pallor may suggest anemia or ↓circulation.

SACRUM • Check for edema and pressure areas in immobilized clients.

NAILS • Cyanosis. Clubbing may indicate chronic low O_2 saturation, as in congenital cardiac or pulmonary disease. Thick nails - poor nutrition and impaired O_2 delivery.

LOWER EXTREMITIES • Absence of hair and thin skin are signs of poor circulation.

LEGS/ANKLES/FEET • Check for edema, presence of pulses, ↓ sensation, pressure areas.

C.J. MILLER ©Nursing Education Consultants, Inc.

Cardiac
NursingEd.com

BLOOD FLOW THROUGH THE CARDIAC VALVES

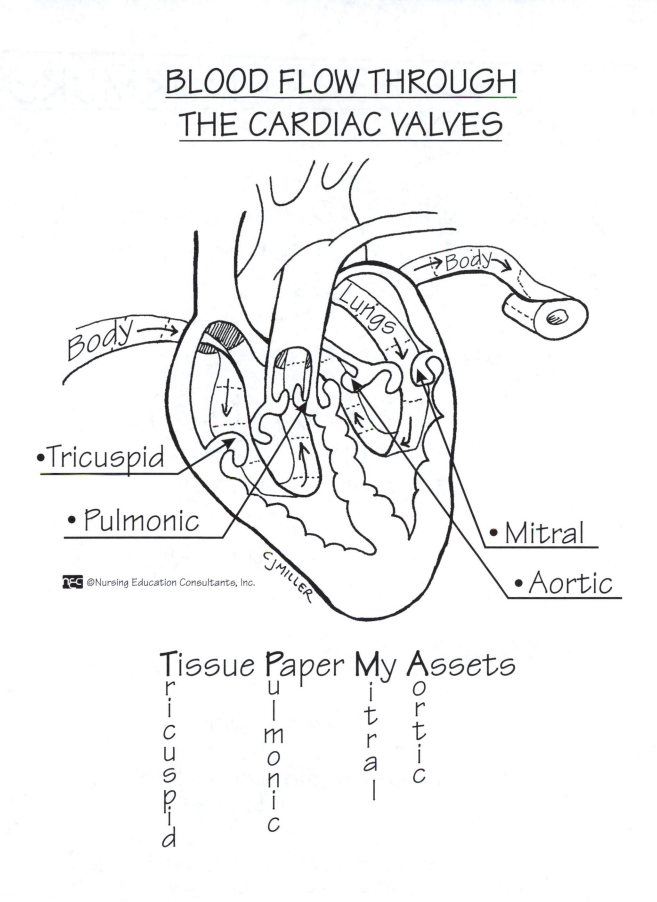

Body →

Lungs ↓

→ Body →

• Tricuspid

• Pulmonic

• Mitral

• Aortic

CJMILLER

Tissue Paper My Assets

Tricuspid Pulmonic Mitral Aortic

HEART MURMURS

Did anyone else hear that... or was it just me?

Causes...(S.P.A.M.S.)
* * Stenosis of a Valve
* * Partial Obstruction
* * Aortic Regurgitation
* * Mitral Regurgitation
* * Septal Defect

Types...

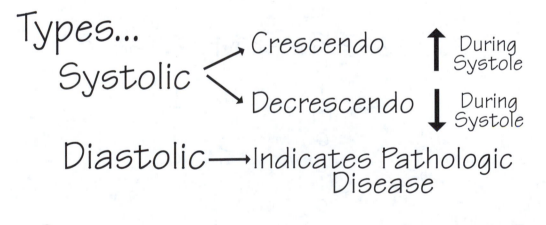

Systolic
- Crescendo — ↑ During Systole
- Decrescendo — ↓ During Systole

Diastolic → Indicates Pathologic Disease

{ Innocent murmurs occur in children or with pregnancy and are noted during systole. }

THE PULMONARY ARTERY CATHETER

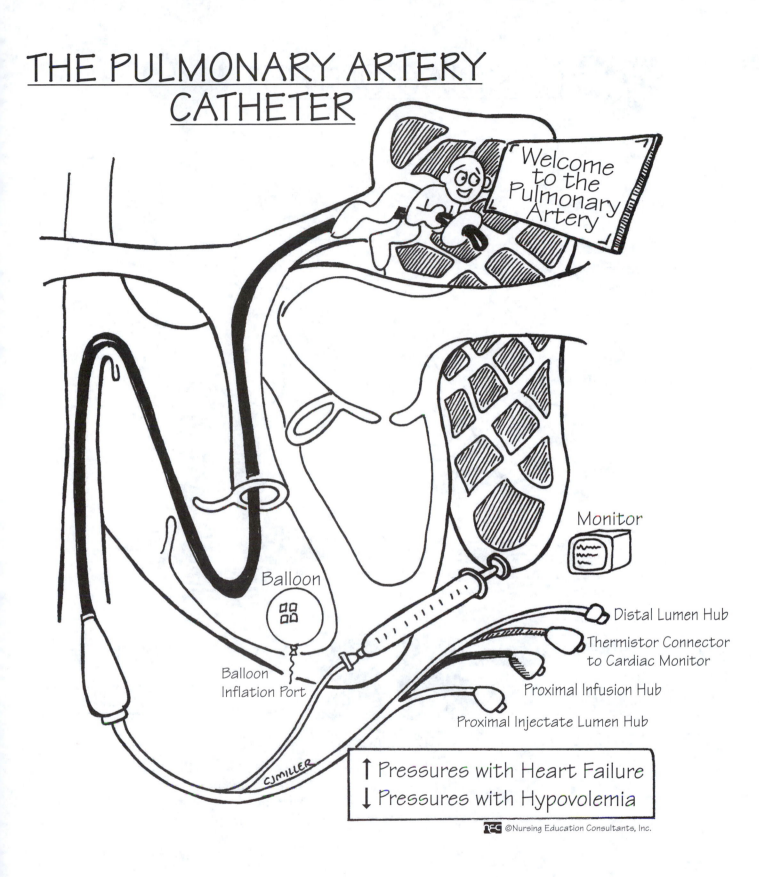

Welcome to the Pulmonary Artery

Balloon

Balloon Inflation Port

Monitor

Distal Lumen Hub

Thermistor Connector to Cardiac Monitor

Proximal Infusion Hub

Proximal Injectate Lumen Hub

CJMILLER

↑ Pressures with Heart Failure
↓ Pressures with Hypovolemia

©Nursing Education Consultants, Inc.

CARDIAC OUTPUT

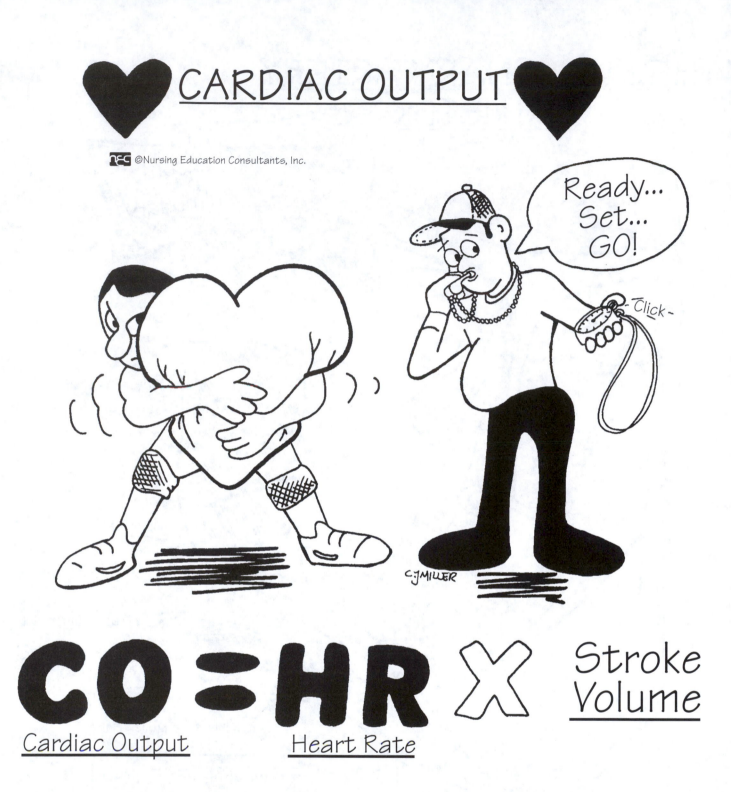

CO = HR X Stroke Volume

Cardiac Output   Heart Rate

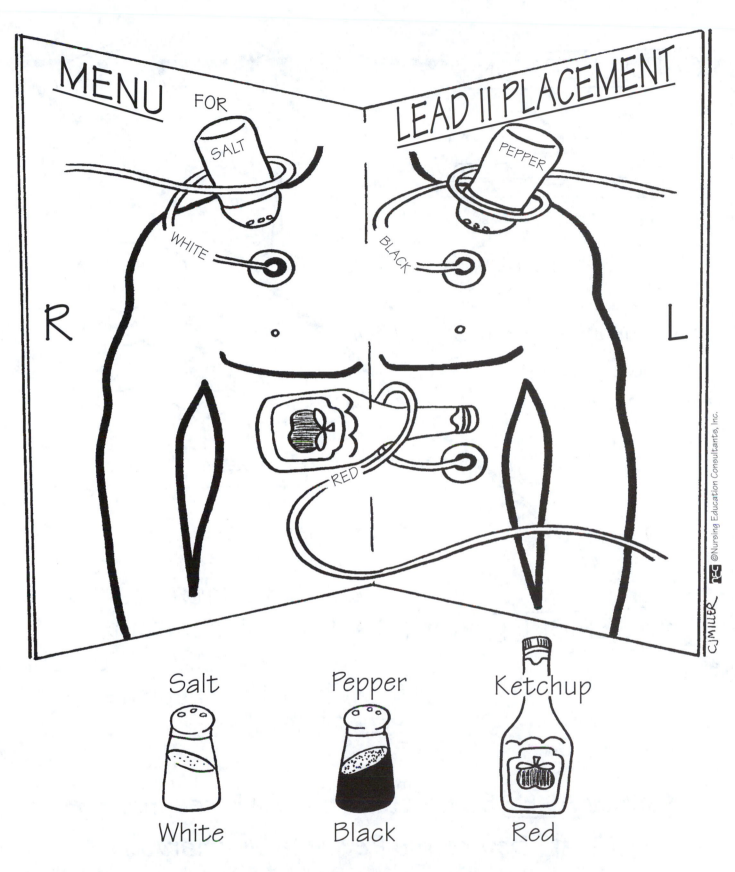

MENU FOR **LEAD II PLACEMENT**

SALT

PEPPER

WHITE

BLACK

R

L

RED

Salt	Pepper	Ketchup
White	Black	Red

"White over right, and smoke (black) over fire (red)."

Cardiac
NursingEd.com

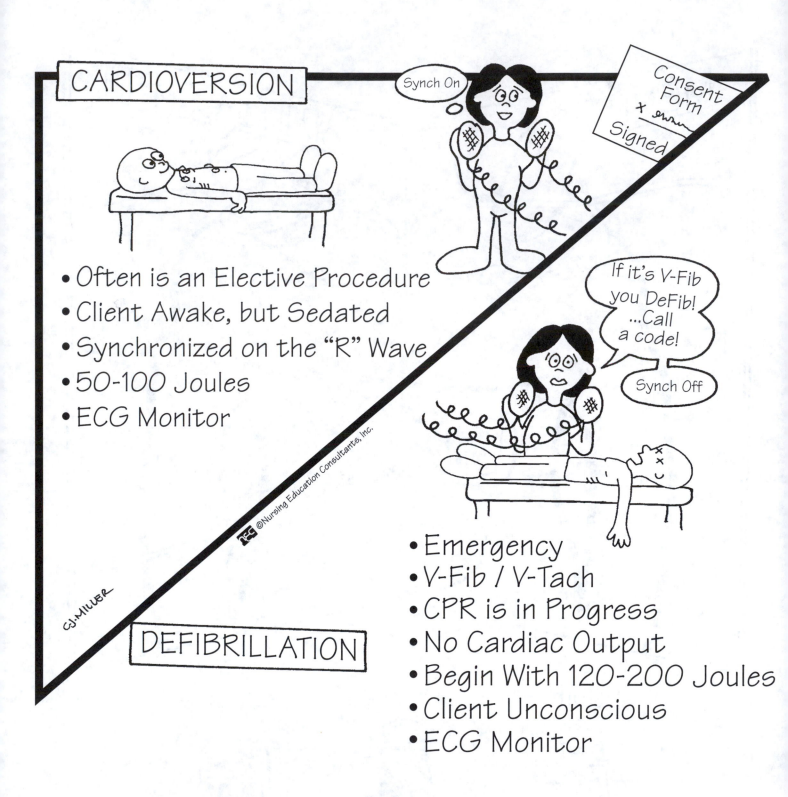

CARDIOVERSION

Synch On

Consent Form X ____ Signed

- Often is an Elective Procedure
- Client Awake, but Sedated
- Synchronized on the "R" Wave
- 50-100 Joules
- ECG Monitor

©Nursing Education Consultants, Inc.

CJ·MILLER

If it's V-Fib you DeFib! ...Call a code!

Synch Off

DEFIBRILLATION

- Emergency
- V-Fib / V-Tach
- CPR is in Progress
- No Cardiac Output
- Begin With 120-200 Joules
- Client Unconscious
- ECG Monitor

<u>Safety Alert:</u> Be Certain That All Personnel Are "Clear" Before The Device Is Discharged.

Cardiac
NursingEd.com

3 AREAS OF DAMAGE AFTER A MYOCARDIAL INFARCTION...

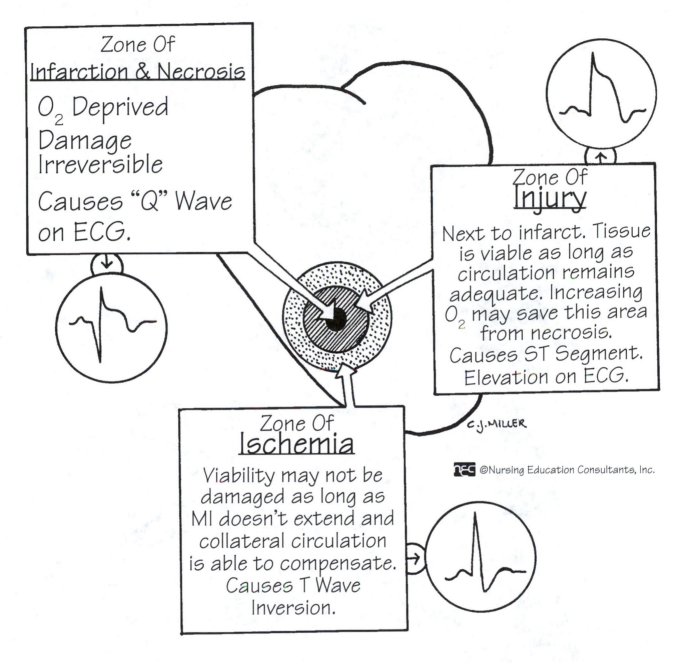

Zone Of Infarction & Necrosis

O_2 Deprived Damage Irreversible

Causes "Q" Wave on ECG.

Zone Of Injury

Next to infarct. Tissue is viable as long as circulation remains adequate. Increasing O_2 may save this area from necrosis. Causes ST Segment. Elevation on ECG.

Zone Of Ischemia

Viability may not be damaged as long as MI doesn't extend and collateral circulation is able to compensate. Causes T Wave Inversion.

C.J. MILLER

IMMEDIATE TREATMENT OF AN M.I.

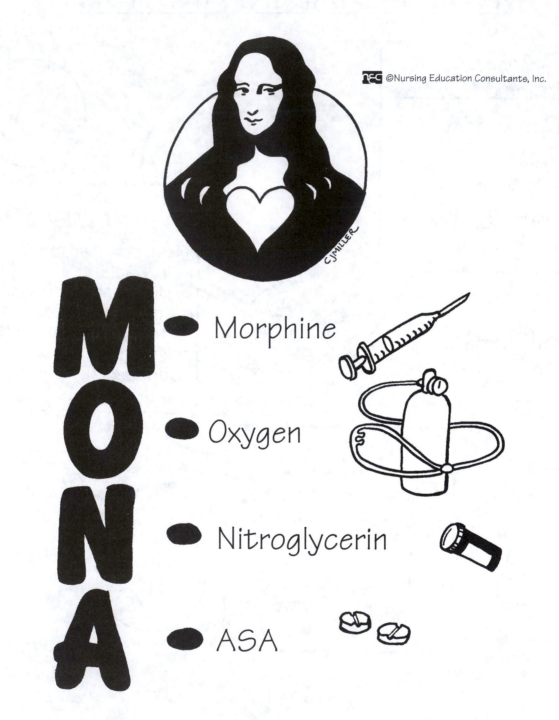

©Nursing Education Consultants, Inc.

M — Morphine

O — Oxygen

N — Nitroglycerin

A — ASA

TREATING CONGESTIVE HEART FAILURE

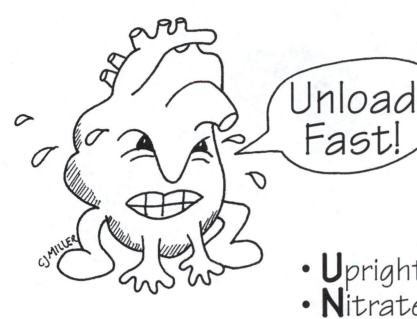

- **U**pright Position
- **N**itrates
- **L**asix
- **O**xygen
- **A**CE Inhibitors
- **D**igoxin

- **F**luids (Decrease)
- **A**fterload (Decrease)
- **S**odium Restriction
- **T**est (Digoxin Level, ABGs, Potassium Level)

APPENDICITIS

- Peak incidence 10-12 years
- Begins as dull, steady pain in periumbilical area...
Progresses over 4-6 hours & localizes to right lower quadrant

- Low grade fever
- Nausea
- Anorexia

- Sudden pain relief may indicate rupture of appendix (Leads to peritonitis)

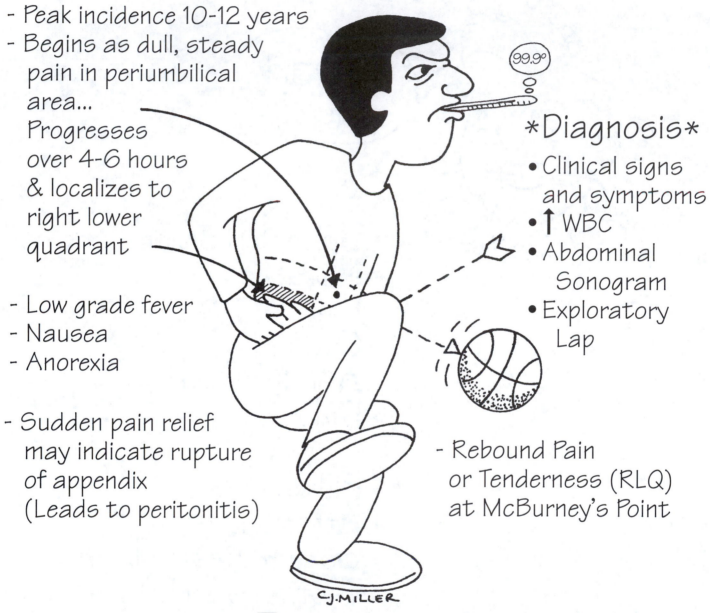

99.9°

Diagnosis
• Clinical signs and symptoms
• ↑ WBC
• Abdominal Sonogram
• Exploratory Lap

- Rebound Pain or Tenderness (RLQ) at McBurney's Point

CJ.MILLER

BOWEL OBSTRUCTION

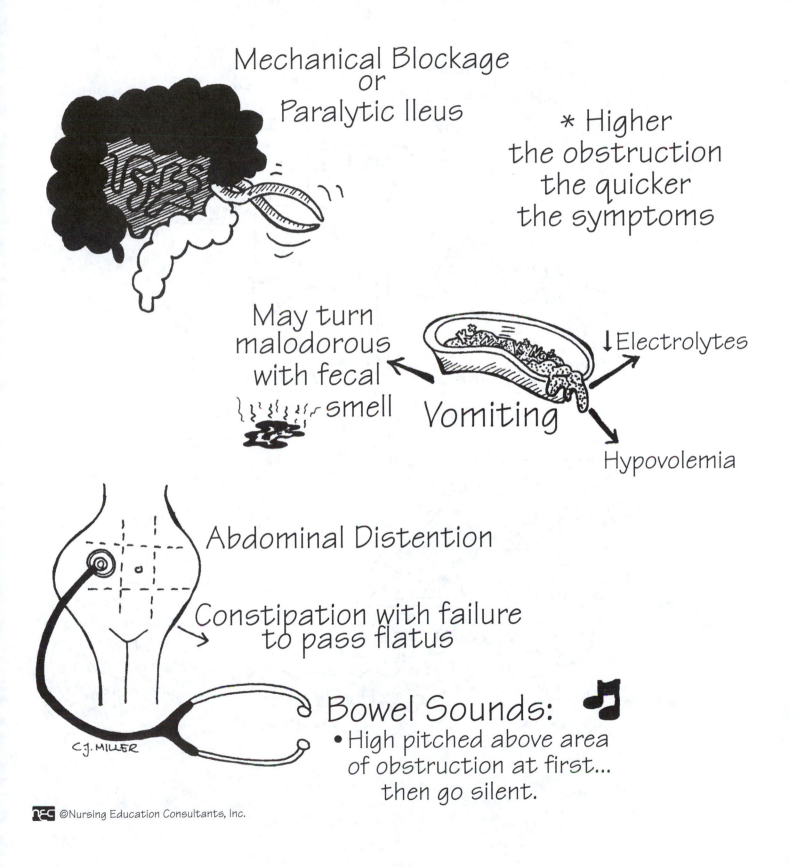

Mechanical Blockage
or
Paralytic Ileus

* Higher
the obstruction
the quicker
the symptoms

May turn
malodorous
with fecal
smell

Vomiting

↓Electrolytes

Hypovolemia

Abdominal Distention

Constipation with failure
to pass flatus

Bowel Sounds:
• High pitched above area
of obstruction at first...
then go silent.

C.J. MILLER

DUMPING SYNDROME

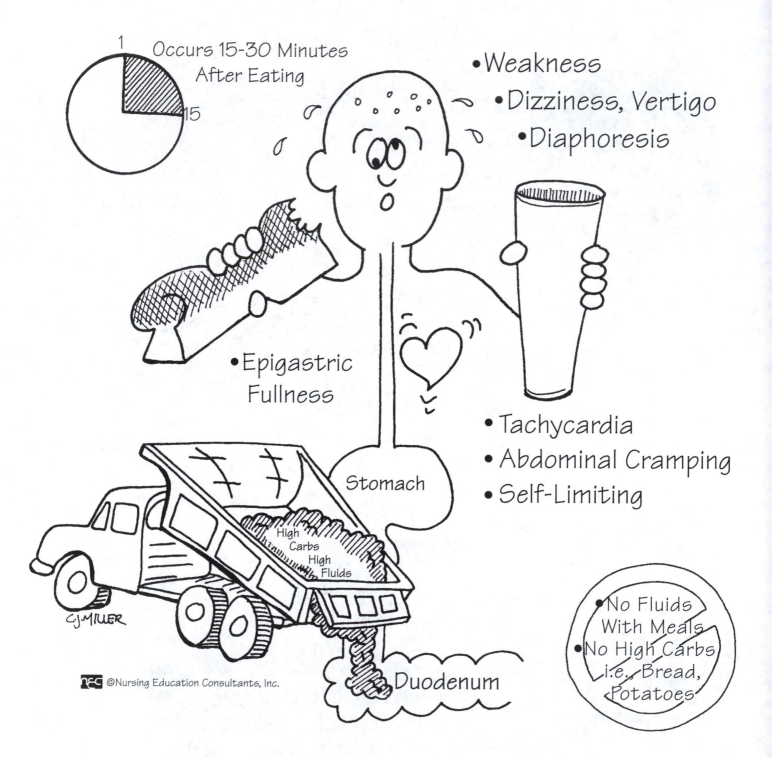

Occurs 15-30 Minutes
After Eating
1
15

- Weakness
- Dizziness, Vertigo
- Diaphoresis

- Epigastric Fullness

- Tachycardia
- Abdominal Cramping
- Self-Limiting

Stomach

High Carbs
High Fluids

Duodenum

- No Fluids With Meals
- No High Carbs i.e., Bread, Potatoes

C.J. MILLER

Gastrointestinal
NursingEd.com

"SIR" HERNIA

Strangulated...

Blood supply is cut off, emergency surgery situation.

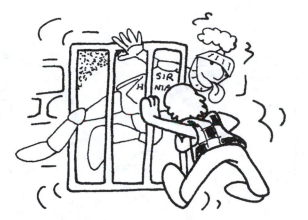

Incarcerated...

Hernia is trapped outside peritoneal cavity.

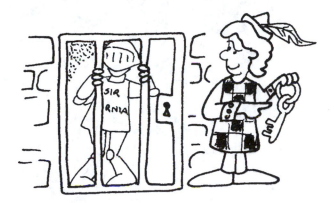

Reducible...

Hernia moves back into peritoneal cavity.

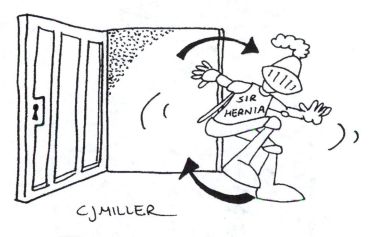

CJ MILLER

©Nursing Education Consultants, Inc.

PERITONITIS

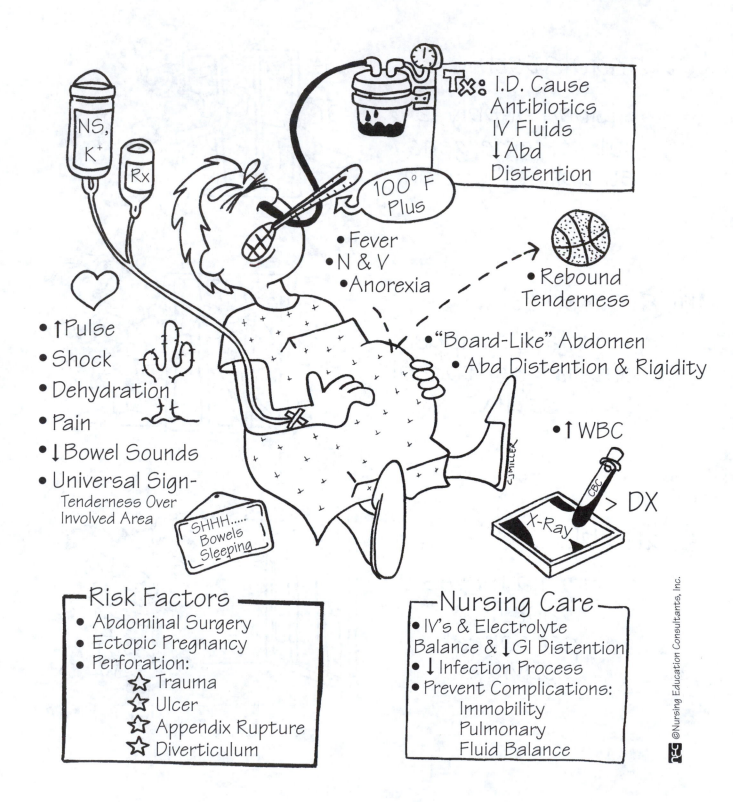

Tx: I.D. Cause
Antibiotics
IV Fluids
↓ Abd
Distention

NS, K⁺

Rx

100° F Plus

• Fever
• N & V
• Anorexia

• Rebound Tenderness

• "Board-Like" Abdomen
• Abd Distention & Rigidity

• ↑ WBC

CBC

X-Ray > DX

• ↑ Pulse
• Shock
• Dehydration
• Pain
• ↓ Bowel Sounds
• Universal Sign-
Tenderness Over
Involved Area

SHHH.....
Bowels
Sleeping

Risk Factors
• Abdominal Surgery
• Ectopic Pregnancy
• Perforation:
   ☆ Trauma
   ☆ Ulcer
   ☆ Appendix Rupture
   ☆ Diverticulum

Nursing Care
• IV's & Electrolyte
Balance & ↓ GI Distention
• ↓ Infection Process
• Prevent Complications:
   Immobility
   Pulmonary
   Fluid Balance

Gastrointestinal
NursingEd.com

HEPATITIS

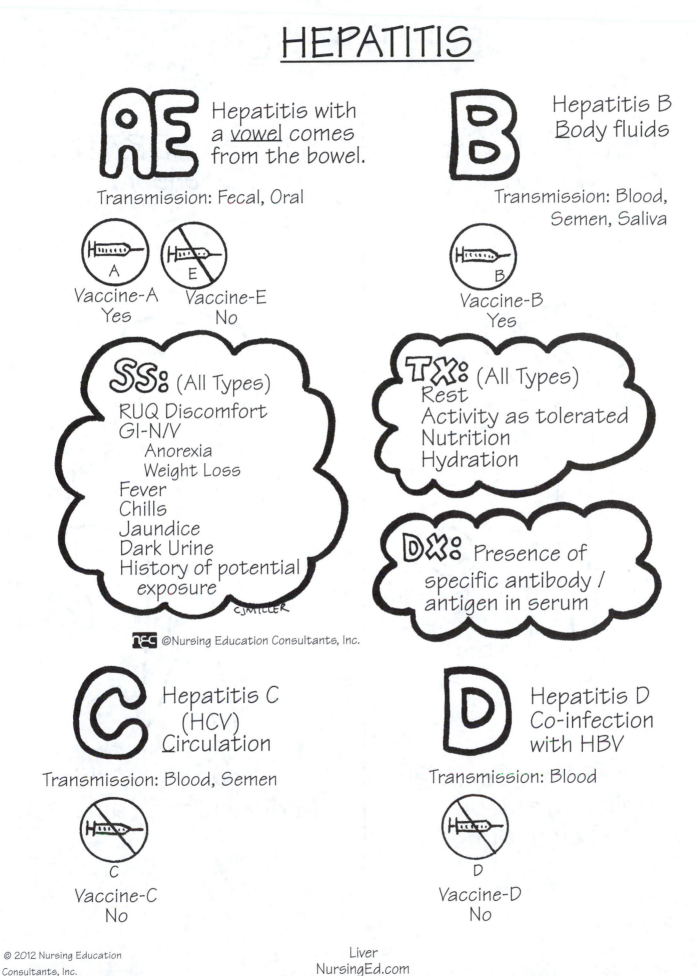

AE Hepatitis with a _vowel_ comes from the bowel.

Transmission: Fecal, Oral

Vaccine-A Yes

Vaccine-E No

B Hepatitis B
_B_ody fluids

Transmission: Blood, Semen, Saliva

Vaccine-B Yes

SS: (All Types)
RUQ Discomfort
GI-N/V
   Anorexia
   Weight Loss
Fever
Chills
Jaundice
Dark Urine
History of potential
   exposure

CJMILLER

©Nursing Education Consultants, Inc.

TX: (All Types)
Rest
Activity as tolerated
Nutrition
Hydration

DX: Presence of specific antibody / antigen in serum

C Hepatitis C
(HCV)
_C_irculation

Transmission: Blood, Semen

Vaccine-C No

D Hepatitis D
Co-infection with HBV

Transmission: Blood

Vaccine-D No

POSTURING

DECORTICATE
(Flexor)

DECEREBRATE
(Extensor)

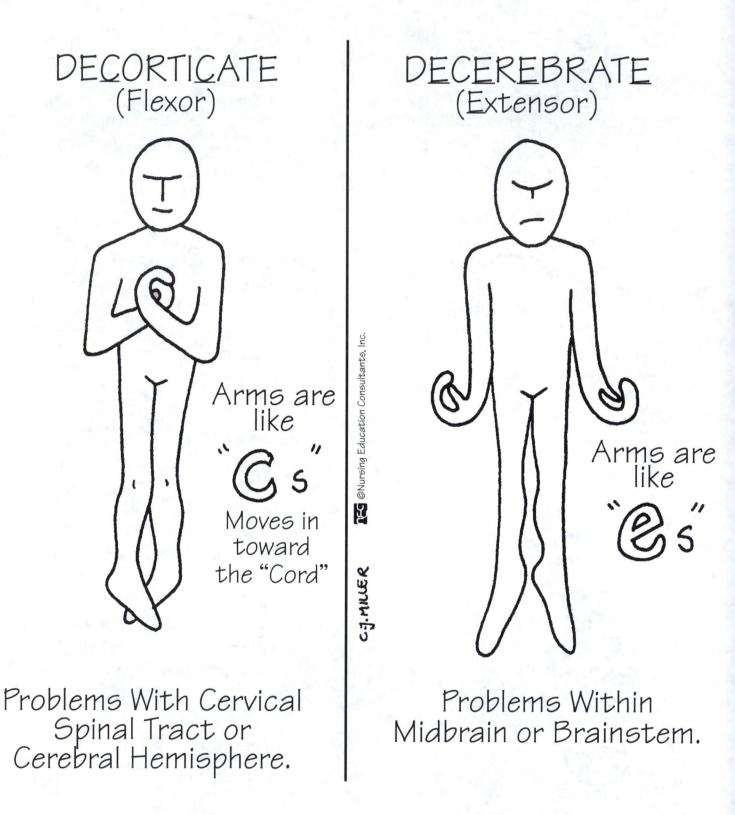

Arms are like

"**C**s"

Moves in toward the "Cord"

Arms are like

"**e**s"

C.J. MILLER

©Nursing Education Consultants, Inc.

Problems With Cervical Spinal Tract or Cerebral Hemisphere.

Problems Within Midbrain or Brainstem.

PARALYSIS

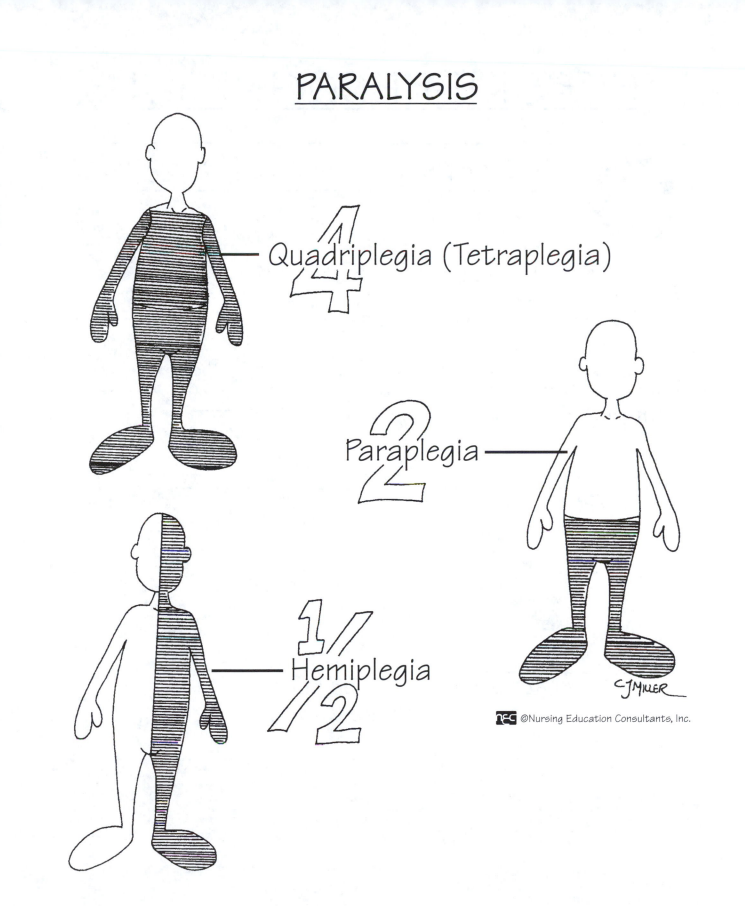

Quadriplegia (Tetraplegia)

Paraplegia

Hemiplegia

©Nursing Education Consultants, Inc.

STROKE RECOGNITION:

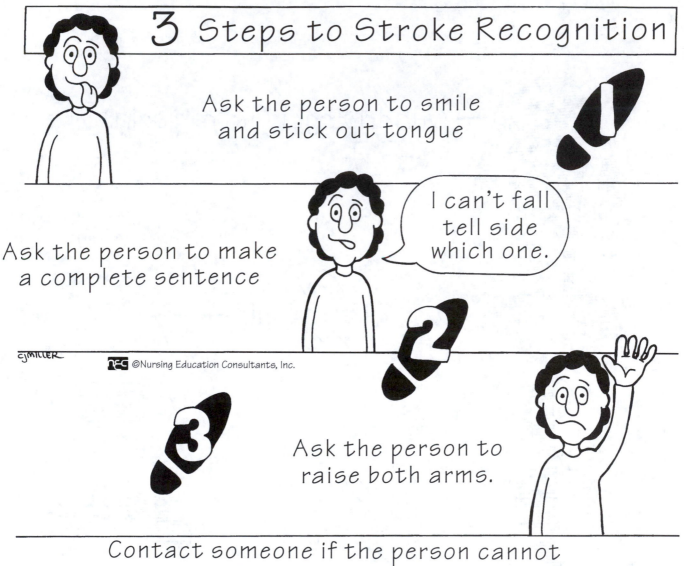

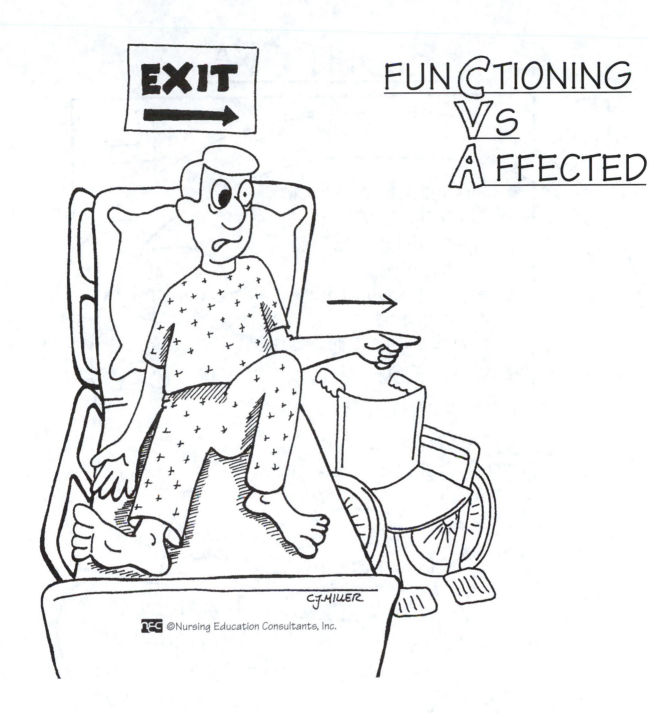

Assist CVA client to get out of bed on the functioning vs affected side.

RIGHT CVA

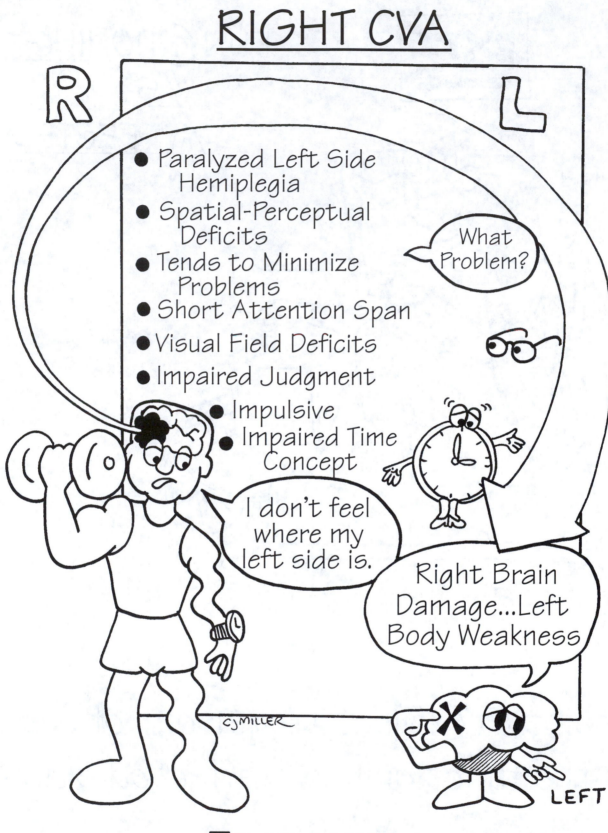

LEFT CVA

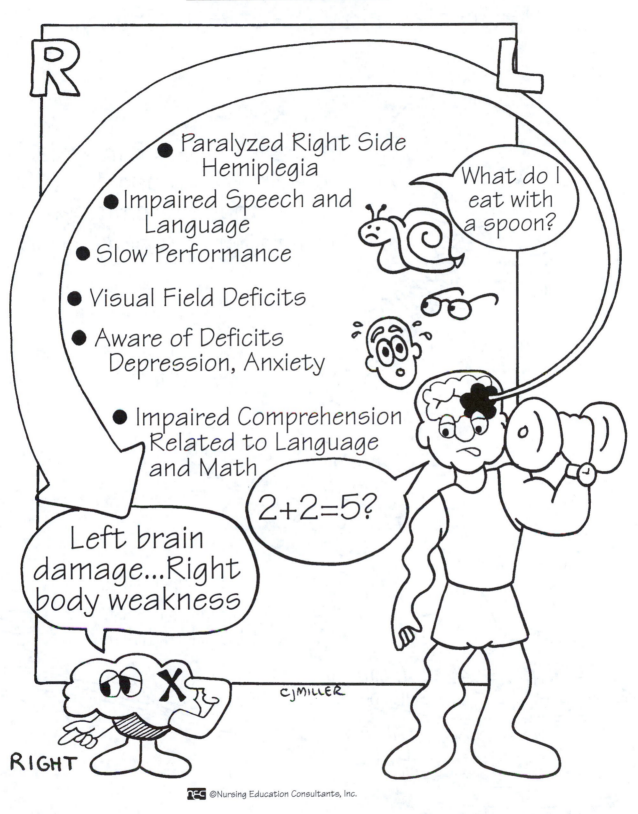

SPINAL CORD INJURY
(Paralysis <u>Below</u> The Level Of Injury)

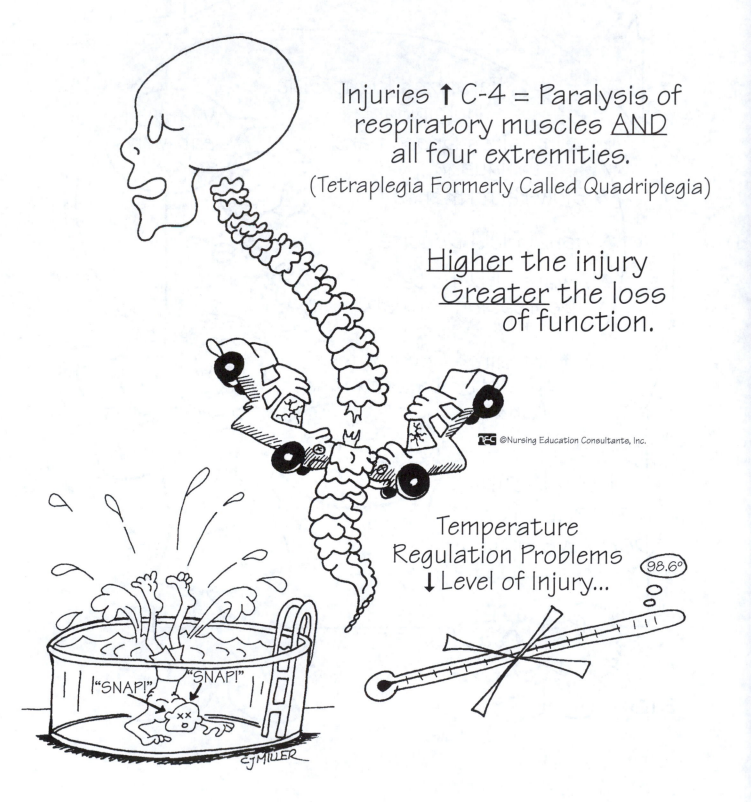

Injuries ↑ C-4 = Paralysis of respiratory muscles <u>AND</u> all four extremities.
(Tetraplegia Formerly Called Quadriplegia)

<u>Higher</u> the injury <u>Greater</u> the loss of function.

Temperature Regulation Problems ↓ Level of Injury...

98.6°

©Nursing Education Consultants, Inc.

"SNAP!" "SNAP!"

CJ MILLER

LEVELS OF SPINAL NERVES

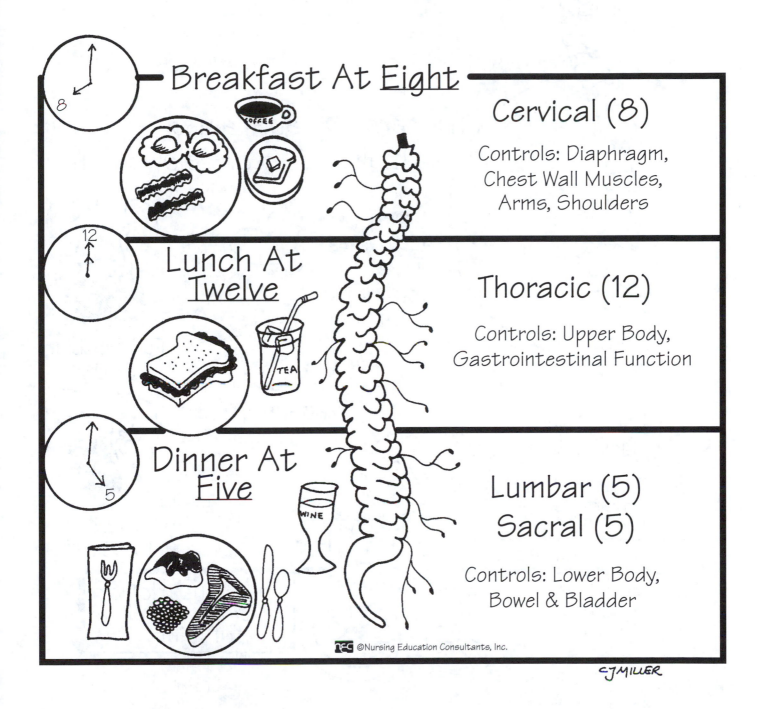

Breakfast At <u>Eight</u>

Cervical (8)

Controls: Diaphragm, Chest Wall Muscles, Arms, Shoulders

Lunch At <u>Twelve</u>

Thoracic (12)

Controls: Upper Body, Gastrointestinal Function

Dinner At <u>Five</u>

Lumbar (5)
Sacral (5)

Controls: Lower Body, Bowel & Bladder

©Nursing Education Consultants, Inc.

CJ MILLER

AUTONOMIC DYSREFLEXIA...
(Spinal Cord Injury At T-6 Or Higher)

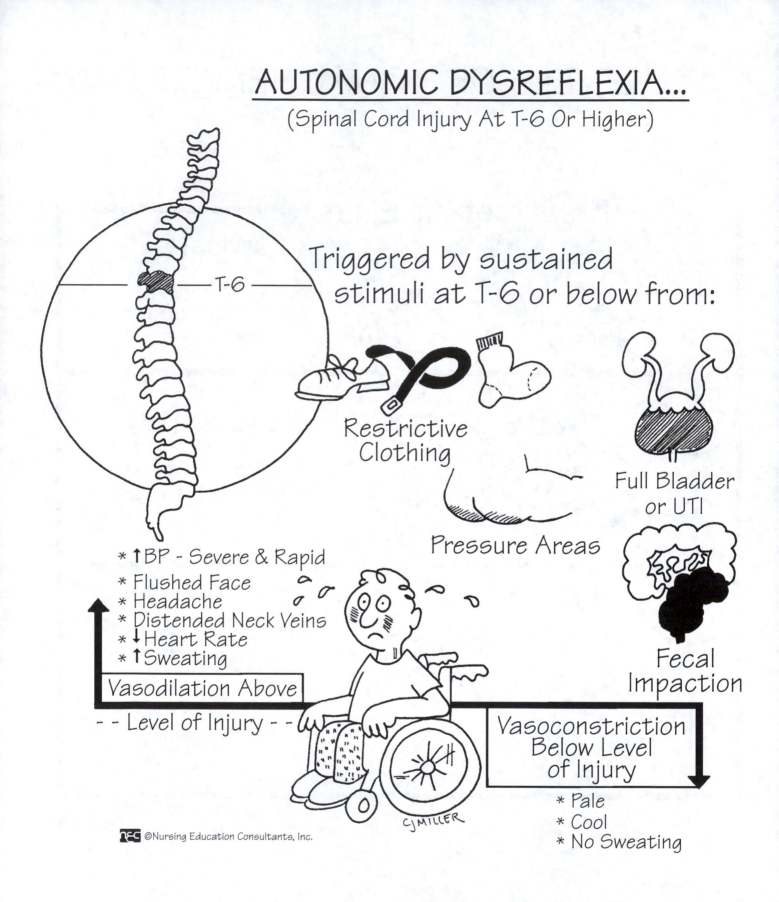

T-6

Triggered by sustained stimuli at T-6 or below from:

Restrictive Clothing

Pressure Areas

Full Bladder or UTI

Fecal Impaction

* ↑BP - Severe & Rapid
* Flushed Face
* Headache
* Distended Neck Veins
* ↓Heart Rate
* ↑Sweating

Vasodilation Above

- - Level of Injury - -

Vasoconstriction Below Level of Injury
* Pale
* Cool
* No Sweating

CJ MILLER

WARNING SIGNS AFTER A HEAD INJURY
(The First 24 Hours)

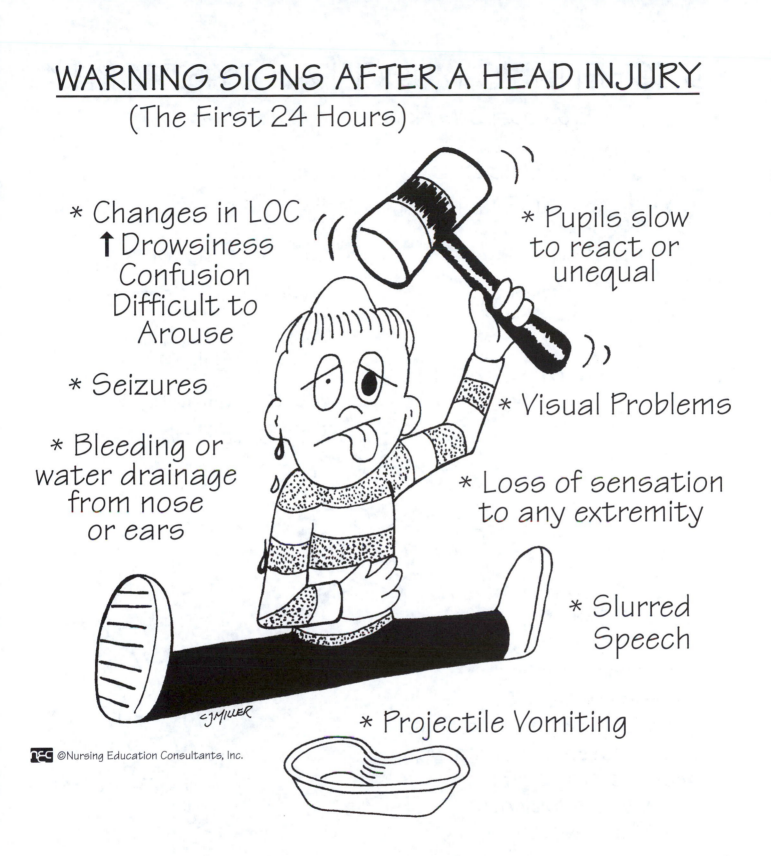

* Changes in LOC
  ↑ Drowsiness
  Confusion
  Difficult to
  Arouse

* Seizures

* Bleeding or
water drainage
from nose
or ears

* Pupils slow
to react or
unequal

* Visual Problems

* Loss of sensation
to any extremity

* Slurred
Speech

* Projectile Vomiting

DUCHENNE'S MUSCULAR DYSTROPHY

* Progressive Weakness & Muscle Wasting *

ONSET 3-5 Years Old

GENETIC ...Primarily Males

- History of motor
  development delay
- Clumsiness
- Frequent falls
- Difficulty climbing stairs,
  running, and riding tricycle

Gower's Sign

- Waddling Gait, Marked Lordosis,
  Large Calf Muscles
- Ambulation frequently
  impossible by age 12.
- As breathing muscles become
  more affected, life-threatening
  infections are common. This
  usually leads to death
  by age 15-18 years.
- Nursing Considerations -
  - Fatigue   • Frequent Infections
  - Mobility   • Psychological Effects   • Maintain Function

Neurology
NursingEd.com

MULTIPLE SCLEROSIS

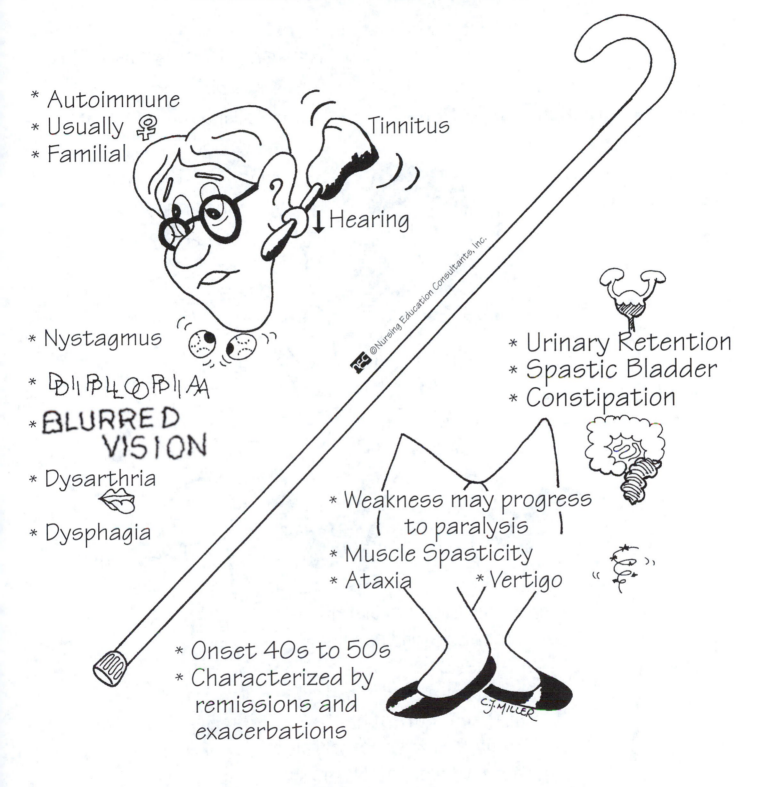

* Autoimmune
* Usually ♀
* Familial

Tinnitus

↓ Hearing

* Nystagmus

* DIPLOPIA

* BLURRED VISION

* Dysarthria

* Dysphagia

* Urinary Retention
* Spastic Bladder
* Constipation

* Weakness may progress to paralysis
* Muscle Spasticity
* Ataxia   * Vertigo

* Onset 40s to 50s
* Characterized by remissions and exacerbations

©Nursing Education Consultants, Inc.

C.J. MILLER

GUILLAIN-BARRÉ SYNDROME

Risk Factors:
- Possibly Autoimmune
- Association with Immunizations
- Frequently preceded by mild respiratory or intestinal infection

- Progresses over hours to days

- Minimal Muscle Atrophy

Causes Problems With:
- Respiration
- Talking
- Swallowing
- Bowel & Bladder Function

Ventilator

O_2

E-T Tube

©Nursing Education Consultants, Inc.
CJ. MILLER

- Symmetrical Paralysis

Begins in lower extremities and ascends bilaterally =
1) Weakness
2) Hypotonia and Areflexia
3) Bilateral Paresthesia Progressing to Paralysis
4) Pain - Worse at Night
5) Autonomic Disturbances - ↑BP, ↓Pulse, Heart Block

TETANUS
(Lockjaw)

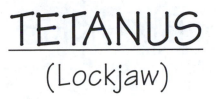

* Intact Sensorium

* Headache

* Difficulty Swallowing

* Irritability

* Tonic Spasms Leading to Laryngospasm

* Prevention - Childhood Immunizations

* Spasms of Facial Muscles
  • Fixed Sardonic Smile
  • Elevated Eyebrows

* Jaw Stiffness

* Fever

* Restlessness

* Exaggerated Reflexes

* Profuse Sweating

* Progressive Involvement Causes Opisthotonos

J. MILLER

©Nursing Education Consultants, Inc.

SEIZURES

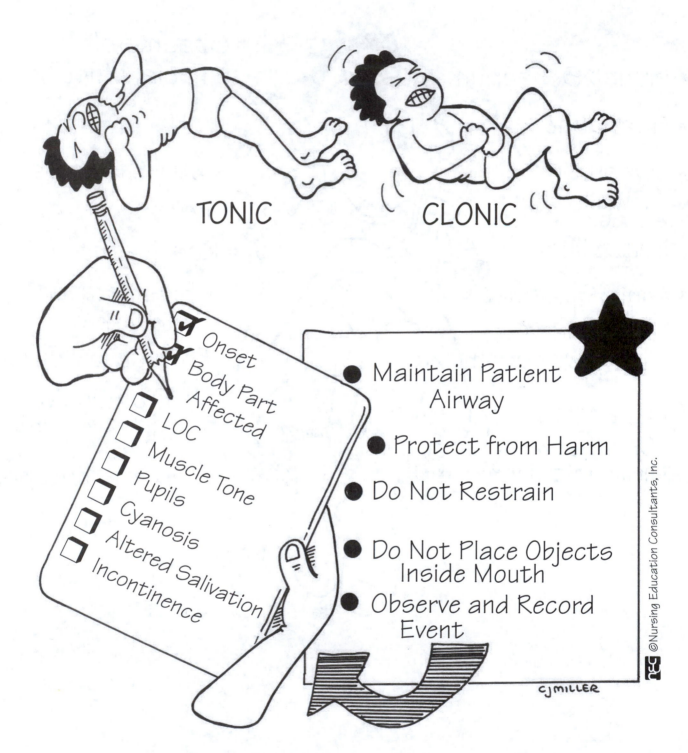

TONIC

CLONIC

- Onset
- Body Part Affected
- LOC
- Muscle Tone
- Pupils
- Cyanosis
- Altered Salivation
- Incontinence

- Maintain Patient Airway
- Protect from Harm
- Do Not Restrain
- Do Not Place Objects Inside Mouth
- Observe and Record Event

CJMILLER

©Nursing Education Consultants, Inc.

Neurology
NursingEd.com

OSTEOPOROSIS
(After Menopause - ↓Estrogen)

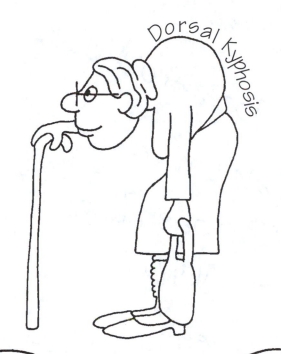

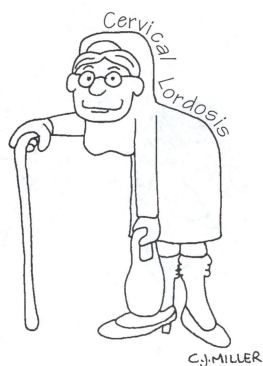

C.J.MILLER

Generalized progressive reduction of bone density, causing weakness of skeletal strength.

Slender, Female, Caucasian, Alcohol Users, Smokers, Steroid Users, Inactive Lifestyles, and Diets Low in Calcium or Vitamin D Deficiency...have the highest risk.

Fractures especially at T-8 & below... Hip & Colles' fractures most common.

OSTEOPOROSIS RISK FACTORS

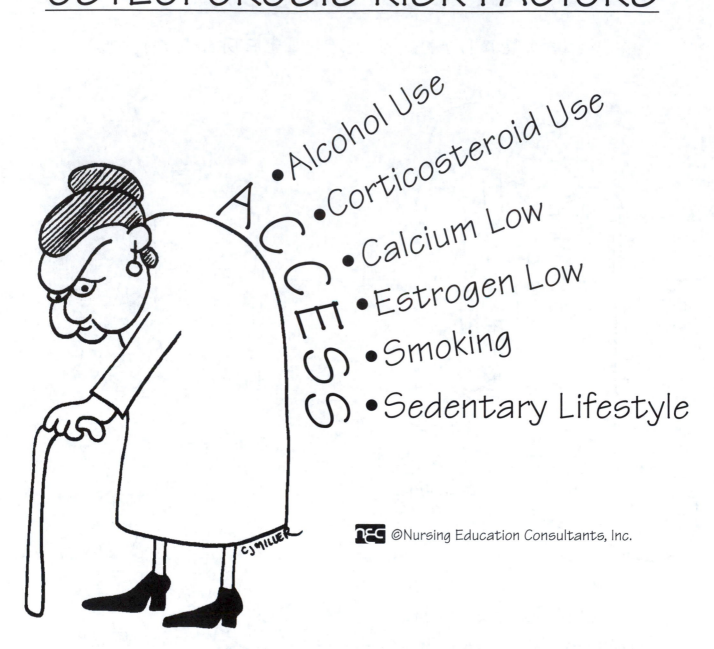

- Alcohol Use
- Corticosteroid Use
- Calcium Low
- Estrogen Low
- Smoking
- Sedentary Lifestyle

A
C
C
E
S
S

©Nursing Education Consultants, Inc.

"Access" (leads to) Osteoporosis

Musculoskeletal
NursingEd.com

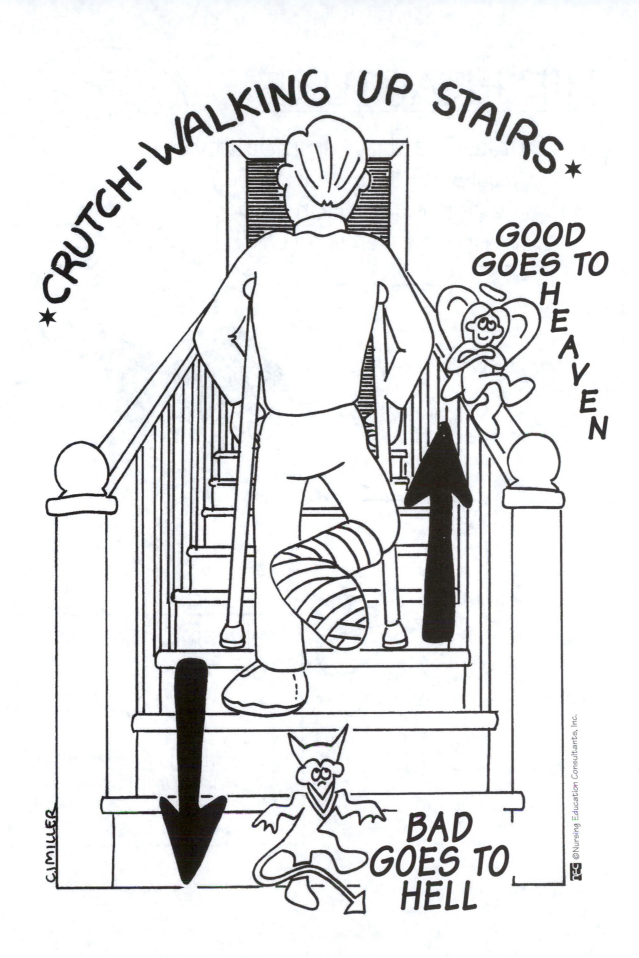

CRUTCH-WALKING UP STAIRS

GOOD GOES TO HEAVEN

BAD GOES TO HELL

HIP FRACTURE

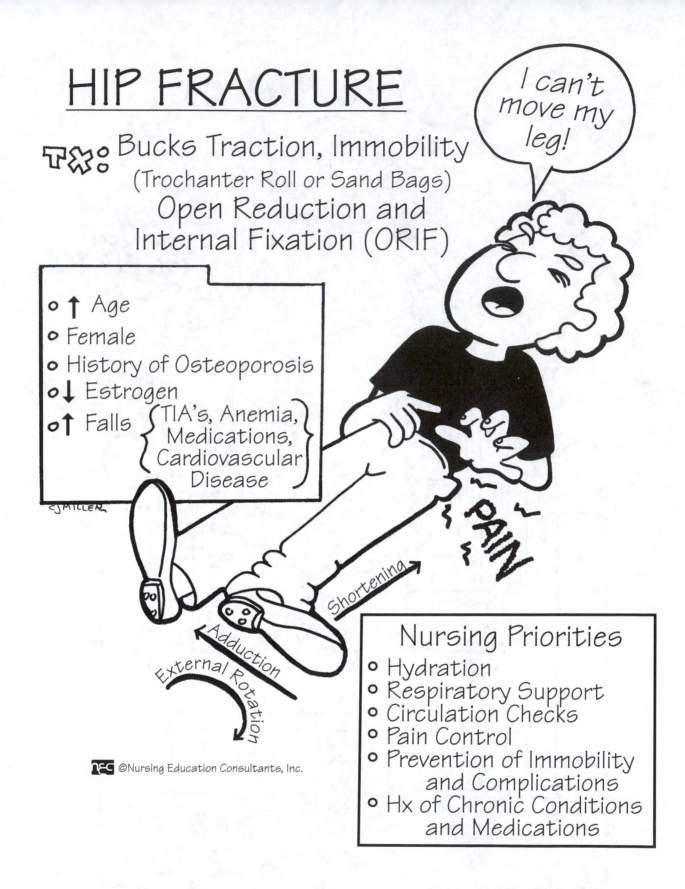

TX: Bucks Traction, Immobility
(Trochanter Roll or Sand Bags)
Open Reduction and
Internal Fixation (ORIF)

I can't move my leg!

- ↑ Age
- Female
- History of Osteoporosis
- ↓ Estrogen
- ↑ Falls { TIA's, Anemia, Medications, Cardiovascular Disease }

CJMILLER

Shortening

PAIN

Adduction

External Rotation

Nursing Priorities
- Hydration
- Respiratory Support
- Circulation Checks
- Pain Control
- Prevention of Immobility and Complications
- Hx of Chronic Conditions and Medications

©Nursing Education Consultants, Inc.

Musculoskeletal
NursingEd.com

POST-OP CARE
HIP FRACTURES

Nursing Care

- Cough / Deep Breath Q 2°
- Stockings & Compression Devices to ↓ DVT, Venous Stasis
- Turn q2h, Maintain Leg Abduction (Wedge Pillow)
- Circulation & Neuro Status ✓'s of Affected Leg
- Pain Control
- Out of the Bed First Postoperative Day
- ✓ Under Client/Dressing for Drainage

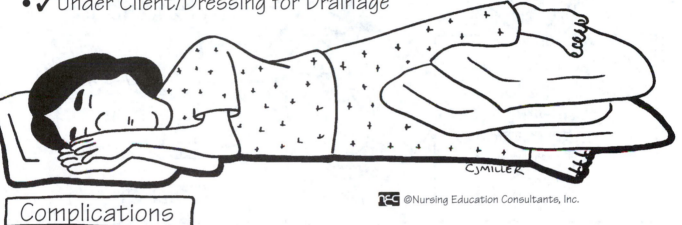

©Nursing Education Consultants, Inc.

Complications

- Prosthesis Dislocation
- DVT
- Neurovascular Complications
  (Bleeding, Swelling, Compartment Syndrome)
- Pulmonary Complications (Atelectasis)
- Urinary Retention
- Delayed Complications (Infection, Nonunion)

 Watch For
- Severe Pain
- Inability to Move Leg
  & Lump in Buttock
- Limb Shortening
  & External Rotation

GLOMERULONEPHRITIS

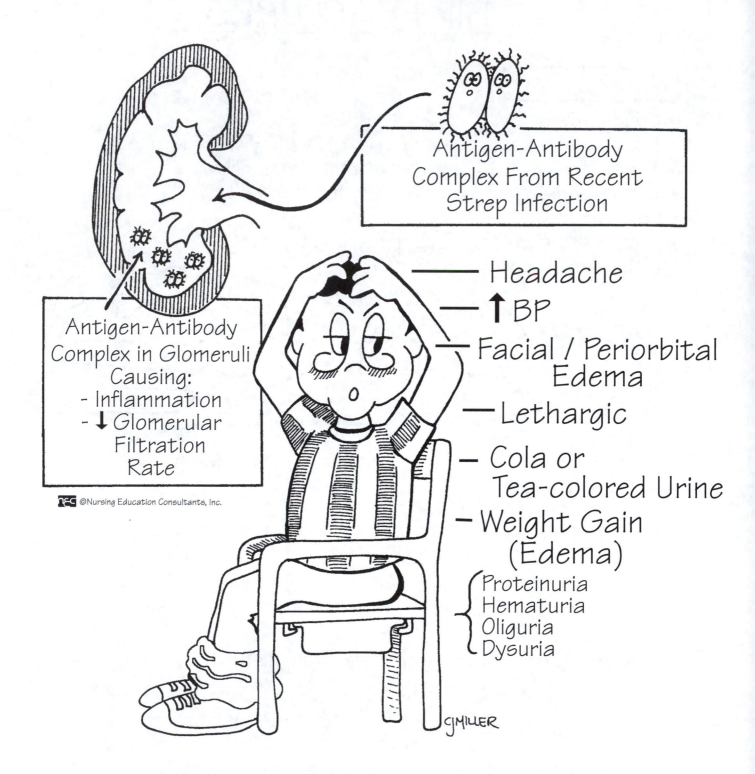

Antigen-Antibody Complex From Recent Strep Infection

Antigen-Antibody Complex in Glomeruli Causing:
- Inflammation
- ↓ Glomerular Filtration Rate

©Nursing Education Consultants, Inc.

Headache

↑ BP

Facial / Periorbital Edema

Lethargic

Cola or Tea-colored Urine

Weight Gain (Edema)

Proteinuria
Hematuria
Oliguria
Dysuria

CJMILLER

PREVENTING CYSTITIS

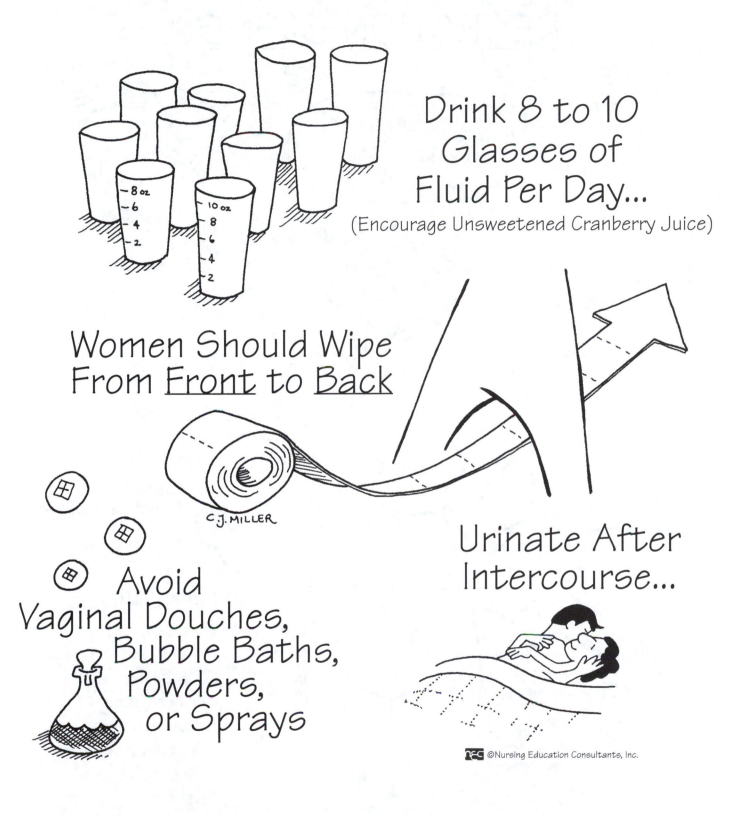

Drink 8 to 10 Glasses of Fluid Per Day...
(Encourage Unsweetened Cranberry Juice)

Women Should Wipe From Front to Back

C.J. MILLER

Avoid Vaginal Douches, Bubble Baths, Powders, or Sprays

Urinate After Intercourse...

©Nursing Education Consultants, Inc.

POST KIDNEY TRANSPLANT REJECTION SIGNS

Hey, Don't Go! I Still Need You!

ACUTE...
- 1 Week to 2 Years
- Oliguria, Anuria
- ↑Temp (>37.8°C - 100°F)
- ↑BP
- Flank Tenderness
- Lethargy
- ↑BUN, K, Creatinine
- Fluid Retention
- Not Uncommon to Have at Least One Rejection Episode

HYPERACUTE...
- Onset with 48 hours
- Malaise, high fever
- Graft tenderness
- Organ must be removed to ↓S & S

Sorry Guy. . .

CHRONIC...
- Gradual Over Months to Years
- ↑In BUN, Creatinine
- Imbalances in Proteinuria Electrolytes
- Fatigue
- Irreversible

Renal
NursingEd.com

RENAL COMPENSATION IN SHOCK

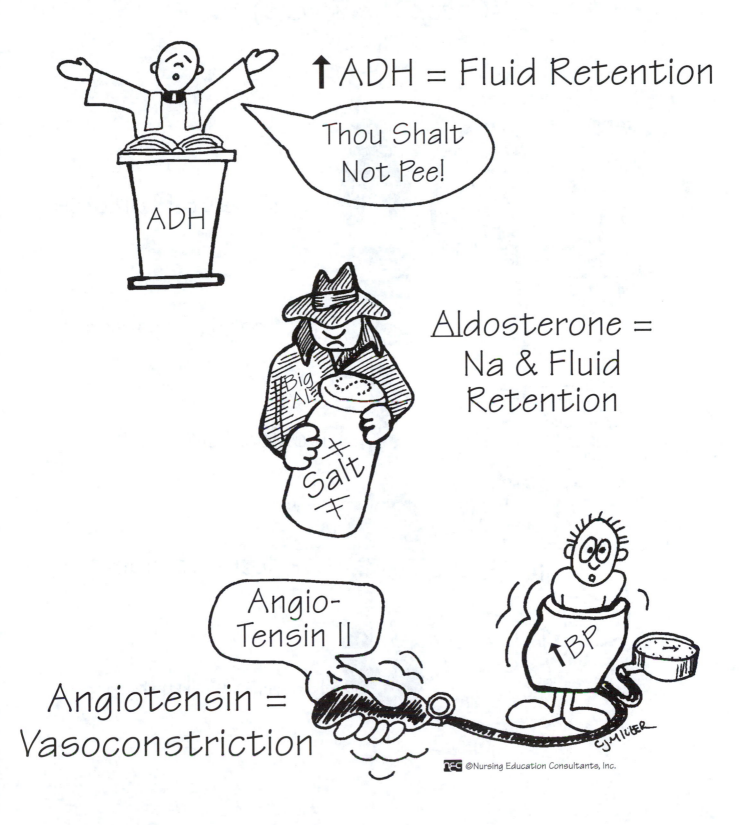

↑ADH = Fluid Retention

Aldosterone = Na & Fluid Retention

Angiotensin = Vasoconstriction

WHO NEEDS DIALYSIS?

(Check The Vowels)

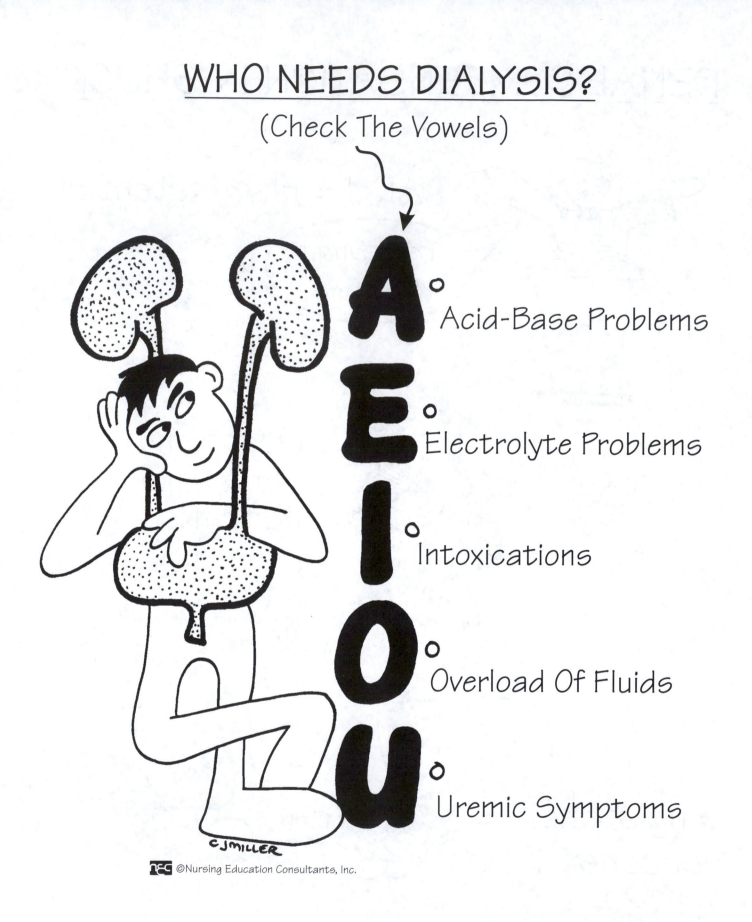

A — Acid-Base Problems

E — Electrolyte Problems

I — Intoxications

O — Overload Of Fluids

U — Uremic Symptoms

Renal
NursingEd.com

PROSTATE PROBLEMS ARE NO...

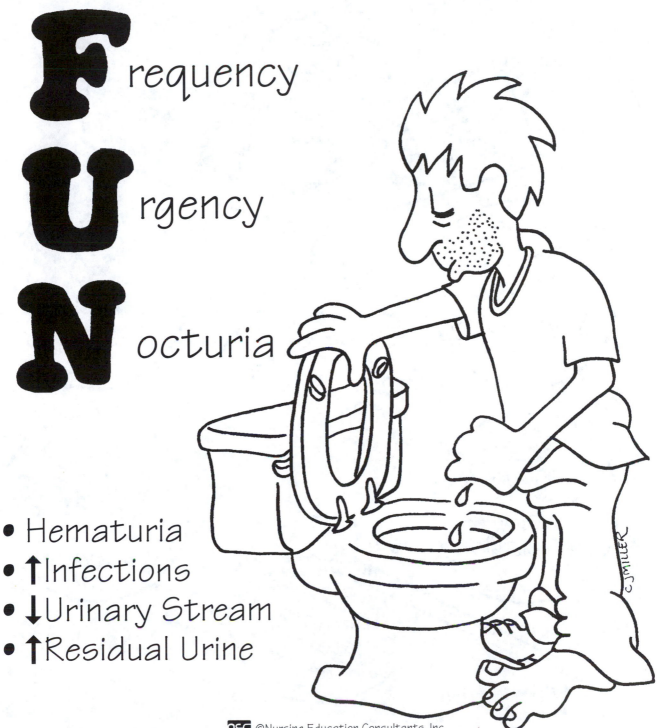

Frequency

Urgency

Nocturia

- Hematuria
- ↑ Infections
- ↓ Urinary Stream
- ↑ Residual Urine

MALIGNANT MELANOMA
(SIGNS OF)

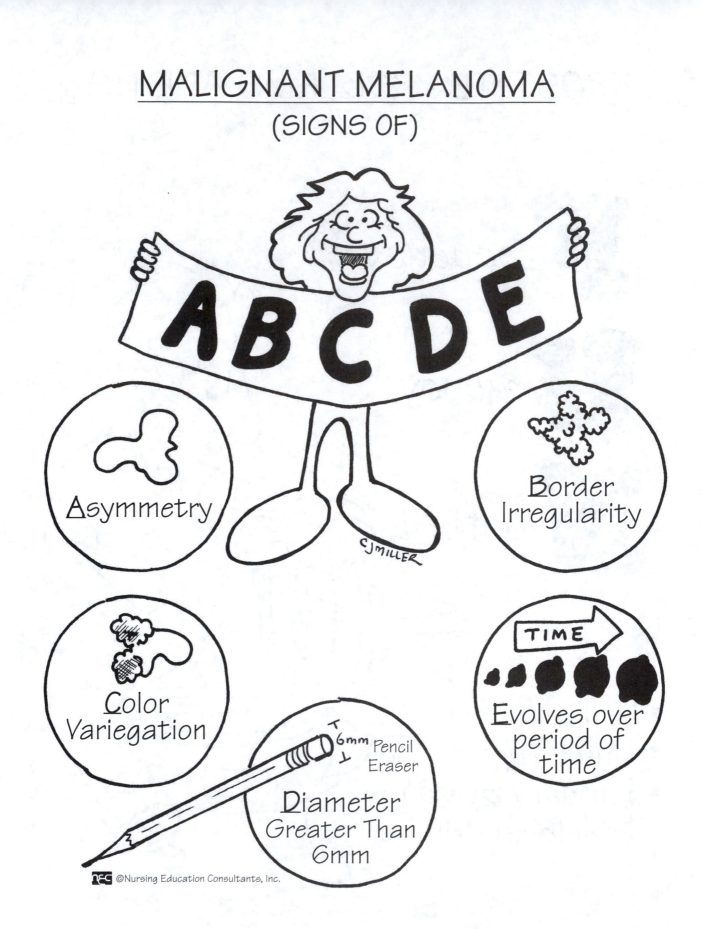

Asymmetry

Border Irregularity

Color Variegation

6mm Pencil Eraser

Diameter Greater Than 6mm

TIME

Evolves over period of time

CJMILLER

Integumentary
NursingEd.com

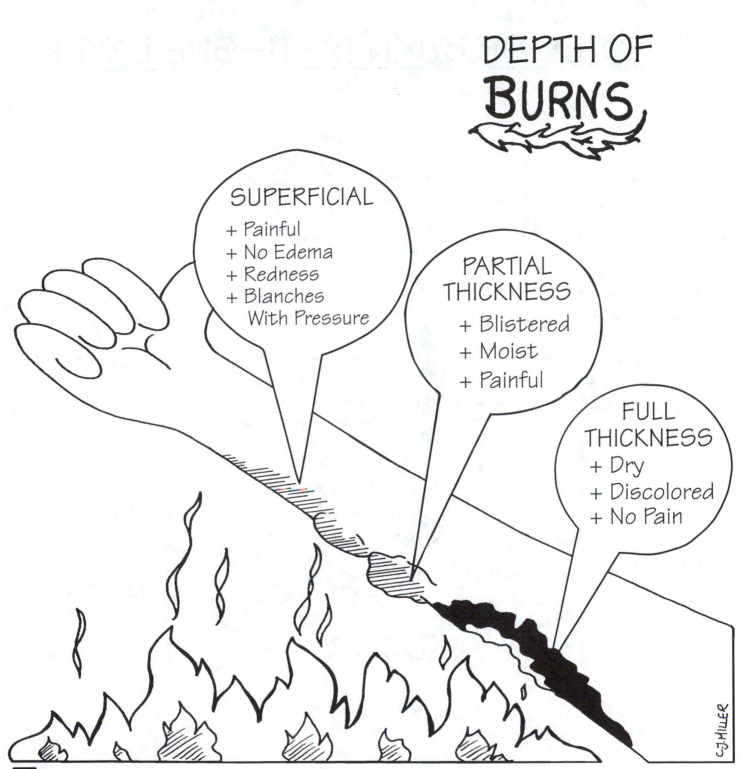

DEGREE OF BURN BY TISSUE LAYER

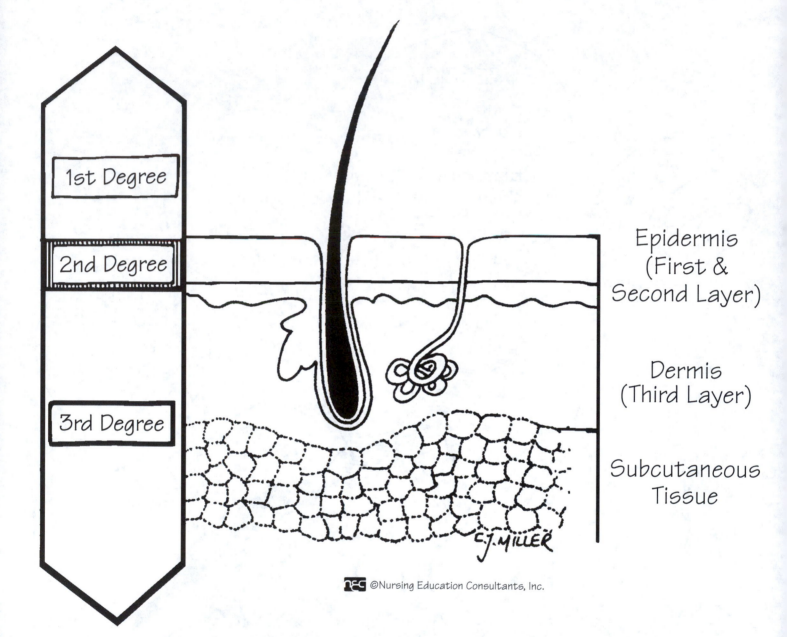

1st Degree

2nd Degree

3rd Degree

Epidermis
(First &
Second Layer)

Dermis
(Third Layer)

Subcutaneous
Tissue

C.J. MILLER

©Nursing Education Consultants, Inc.

Integumentary
NursingEd.com

TIPS ON HEALING SKIN LESIONS

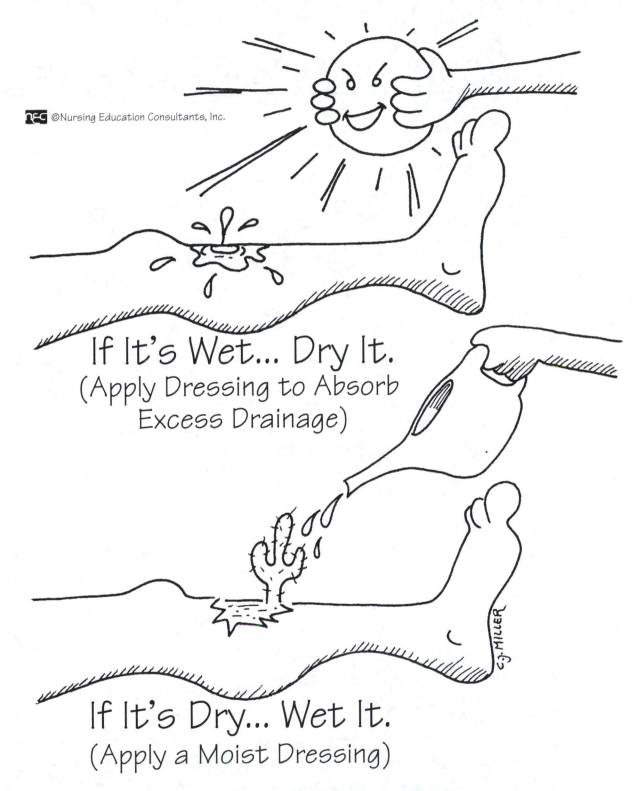

©Nursing Education Consultants, Inc.

If It's Wet... Dry It.
(Apply Dressing to Absorb Excess Drainage)

If It's Dry... Wet It.
(Apply a Moist Dressing)

Note: To promote healing, use a dressing that will continuously provide a moist environment. Wet-to-dry dressings are only for debridement.

Integumentary
NursingEd.com

ROCKY MOUNTAIN SPOTTED FEVER

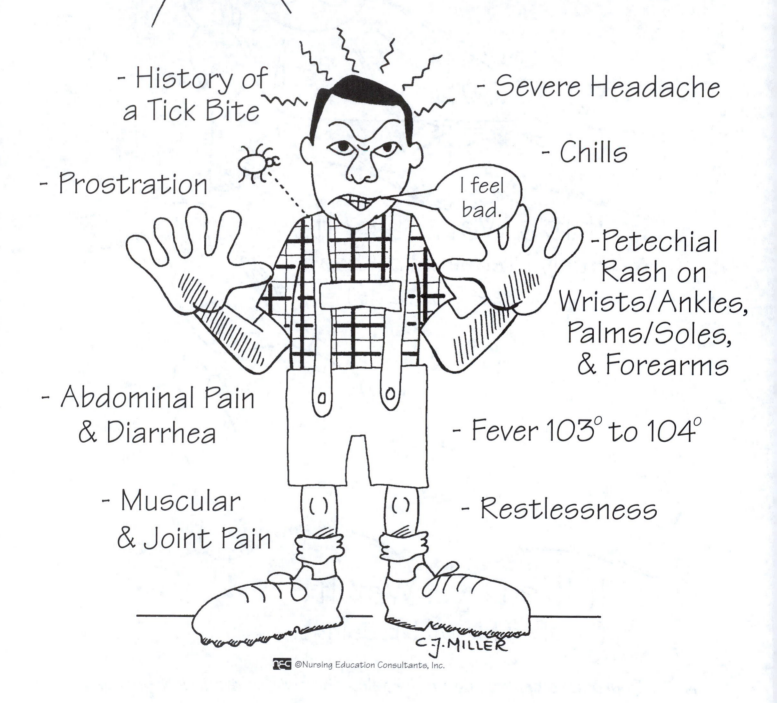

- History of a Tick Bite

- Prostration

- Severe Headache

- Chills

I feel bad.

-Petechial Rash on Wrists/Ankles, Palms/Soles, & Forearms

- Abdominal Pain & Diarrhea

- Fever 103° to 104°

- Muscular & Joint Pain

- Restlessness

C.J. MILLER

LYME DISEASE

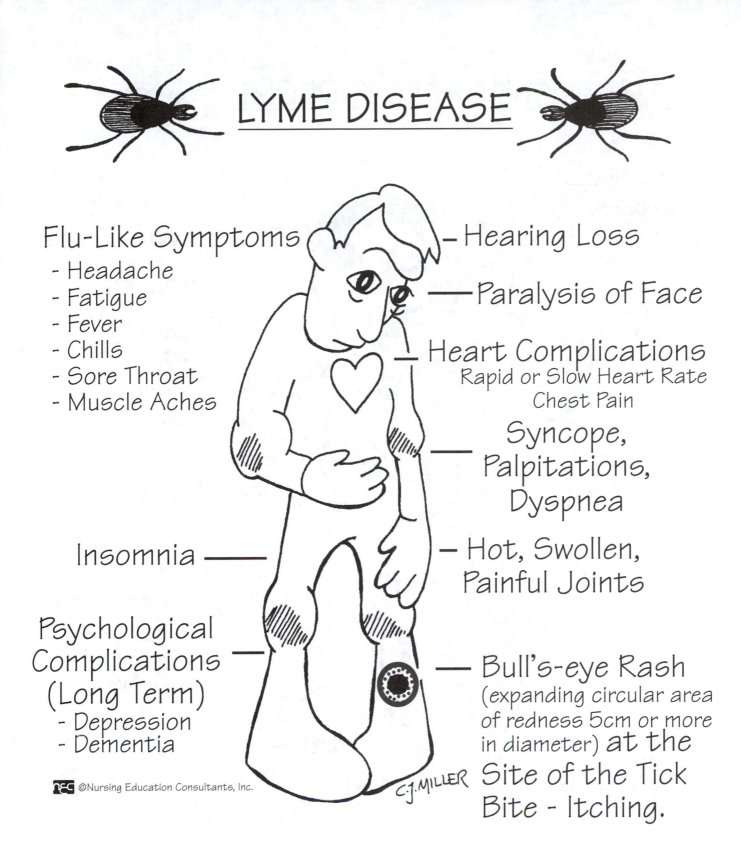

Flu-Like Symptoms
- Headache
- Fatigue
- Fever
- Chills
- Sore Throat
- Muscle Aches

Insomnia

Psychological Complications (Long Term)
- Depression
- Dementia

Hearing Loss

Paralysis of Face

Heart Complications
Rapid or Slow Heart Rate
Chest Pain

Syncope, Palpitations, Dyspnea

Hot, Swollen, Painful Joints

Bull's-eye Rash
(expanding circular area of redness 5cm or more in diameter) **at the Site of the Tick Bite - Itching.**

C.J.MILLER

KAWASAKI SYNDROME

(Acute Systemic Vasculitis)

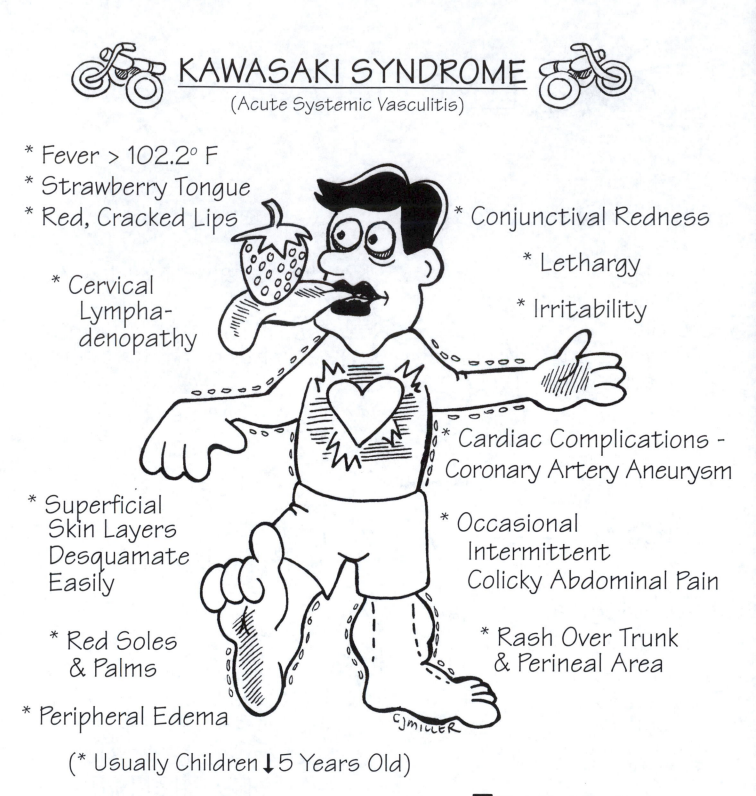

* Fever > 102.2° F
* Strawberry Tongue
* Red, Cracked Lips

* Cervical Lympha-denopathy

* Conjunctival Redness

* Lethargy

* Irritability

* Cardiac Complications - Coronary Artery Aneurysm

* Superficial Skin Layers Desquamate Easily

* Occasional Intermittent Colicky Abdominal Pain

* Red Soles & Palms

* Rash Over Trunk & Perineal Area

* Peripheral Edema

(* Usually Children ↓ 5 Years Old)

PERIPHERAL VASCULAR DISEASE (PVD)
ARTERIAL vs VENOUS ULCERS

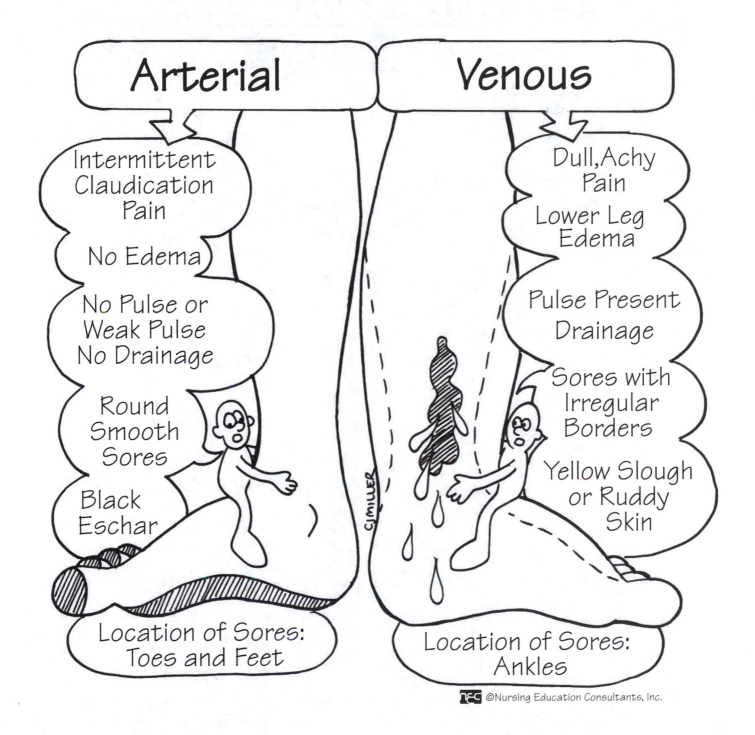

Arterial

Intermittent Claudication Pain

No Edema

No Pulse or Weak Pulse No Drainage

Round Smooth Sores

Black Eschar

Location of Sores: Toes and Feet

Venous

Dull, Achy Pain

Lower Leg Edema

Pulse Present Drainage

Sores with Irregular Borders

Yellow Slough or Ruddy Skin

Location of Sores: Ankles

CJMILLER

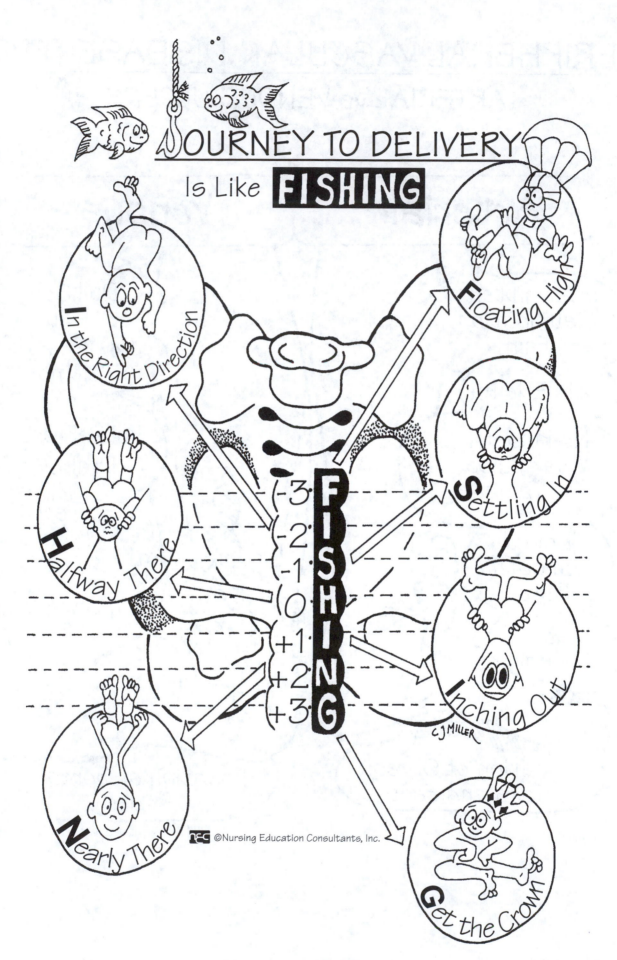

JOURNEY TO DELIVERY

Is Like **FISHING**

In the Right Direction

Floating High

Settling In

Halfway There

FISHING

-3
-2
-1
0
+1
+2
+3

Inching Out

CJ MILLER

Nearly There

©Nursing Education Consultants, Inc.

Get the Crown

CLUE TO CONTRACTIONS

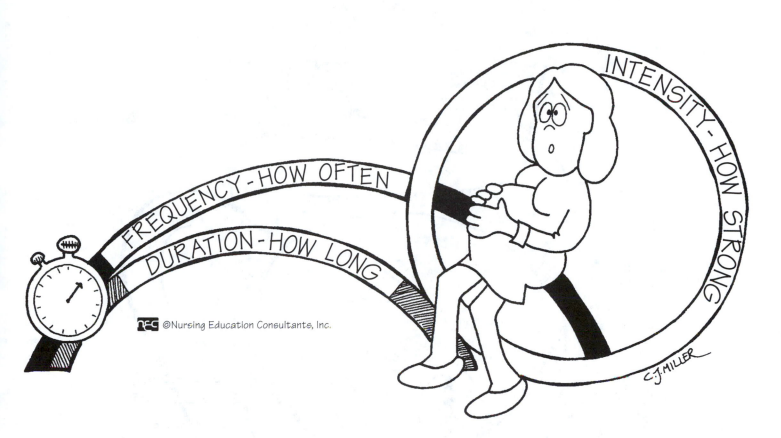

FREQUENCY - HOW OFTEN

DURATION - HOW LONG

INTENSITY - HOW STRONG

@Nursing Education Consultants, Inc.

C.J.MILLER

Can You Figure Out The

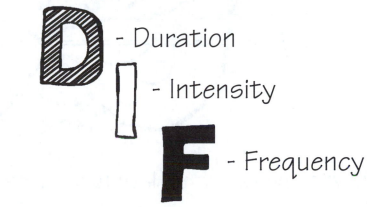

D - Duration

I - Intensity

F - Frequency

FETAL STATION

(Relationship of Fetal Head to Mother's Pelvis)

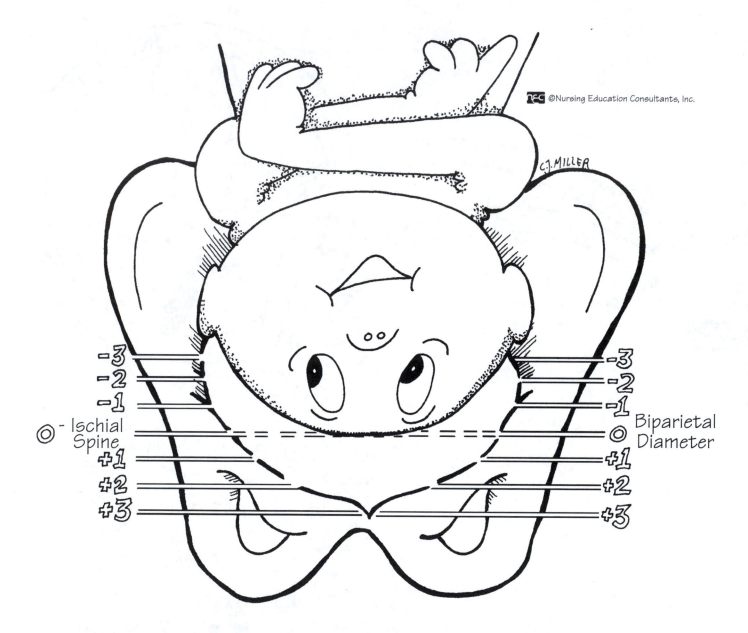

©Nursing Education Consultants, Inc.

C.J. MILLER

-3
-2
-1
◎ - Ischial
Spine
+1
+2
+3

-3
-2
-1
◎ Biparietal
Diameter
+1
+2
+3

I'm At Zero... From Here It's All Positive... I'm On My Way Out!!!

Maternity and Newborn
NursingEd.com

© 2012 Nursing Education
Consultants, Inc.

EARLY & LATE DECELERATIONS

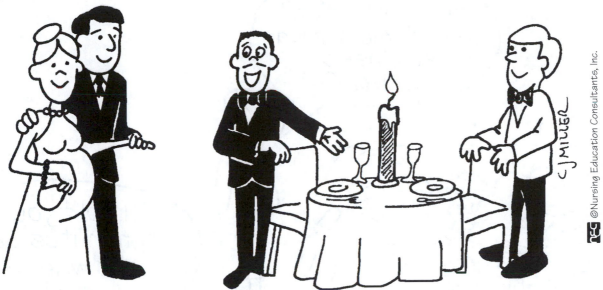

It's okay to be early for dinner...

But don't be <u>late</u>!

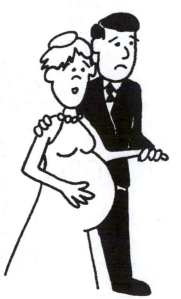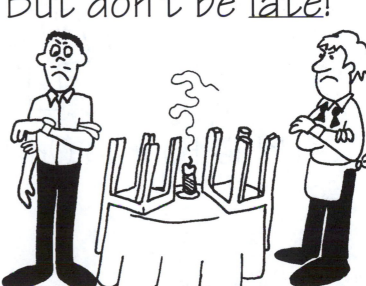

(Late Decelerations Indicate Uteroplacental Insufficiency)

+4 STATION AND DELIVERY

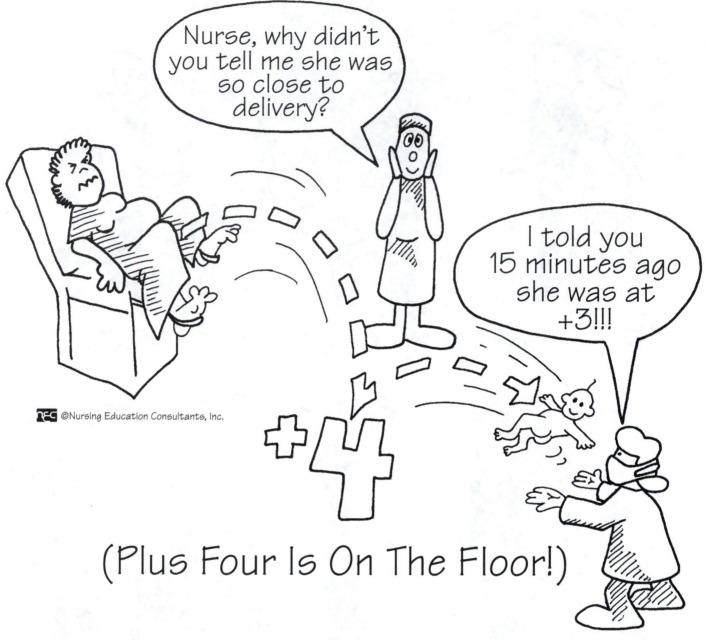

(Plus Four Is On The Floor!)

© 2012 Nursing Education
Consultants, Inc.

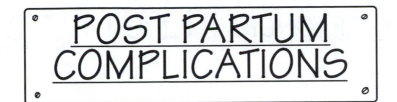

POST PARTUM COMPLICATIONS

RISK FACTORS
Cesarean Delivery
Prolonged ROM
Prolonged Labor
Bladder Catheterization
Hemorrhage
Internal Maternal or
Fetal Monitoring

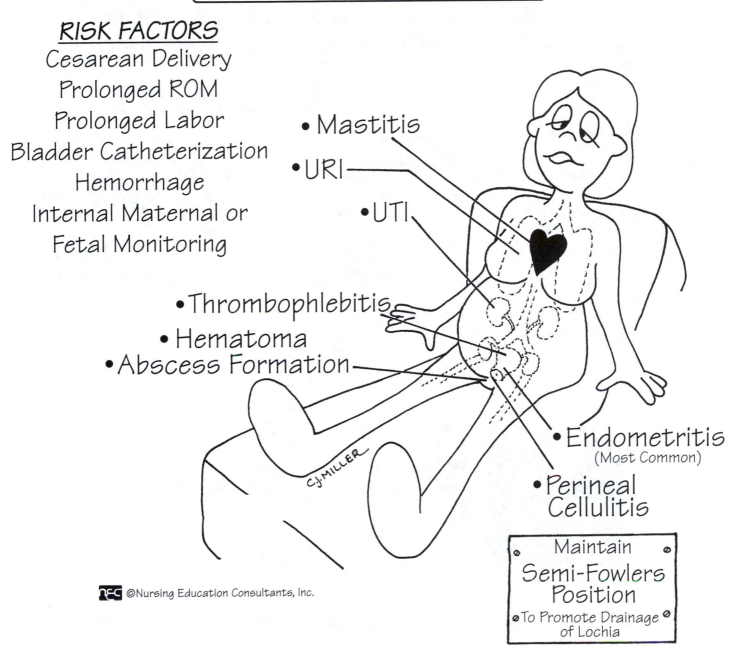

- Mastitis
- URI
- UTI
- Thrombophlebitis
- Hematoma
- Abscess Formation
- Endometritis (Most Common)
- Perineal Cellulitis

Maintain
Semi-Fowlers Position
To Promote Drainage of Lochia

CJ·MILLER

PHENYLKETONURIA (PKU) - Inherited Error In Metabolism

[Toxic levels of Phenylalanine (common protein amino acid) due to inability of body to convert]

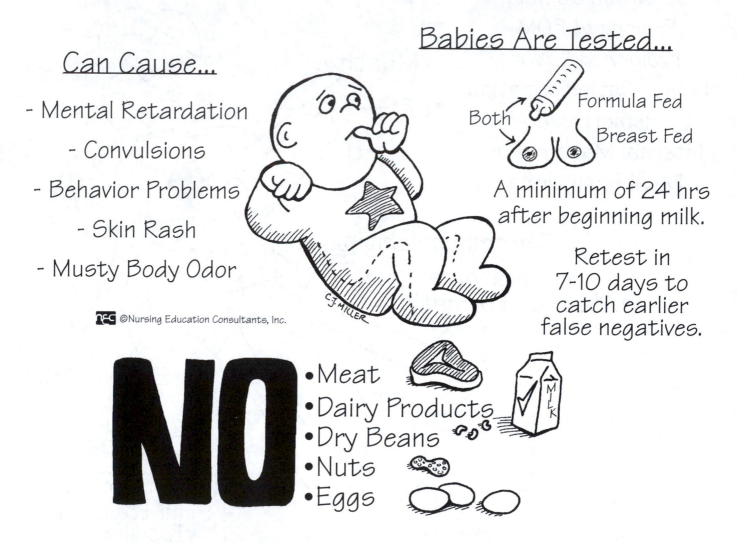

Can Cause...

- Mental Retardation
- Convulsions
- Behavior Problems
- Skin Rash
- Musty Body Odor

©Nursing Education Consultants, Inc.

CJ MILLER

Babies Are Tested...

Both → Formula Fed

Breast Fed

A minimum of 24 hrs after beginning milk.

Retest in 7-10 days to catch earlier false negatives.

NO
- Meat
- Dairy Products
- Dry Beans
- Nuts
- Eggs

MILK

* Cereals, Fruits & Vegetables in Moderation *

Maternity and Newborn
NursingEd.com

© 2012 Nursing Education Consultants, Inc.

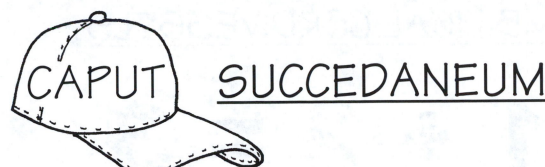

CAPUT SUCCEDANEUM

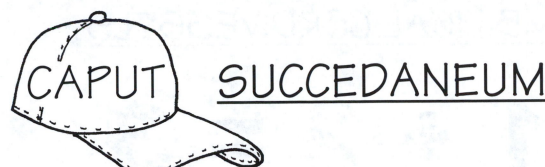
©Nursing Education Consultants, Inc.

Cap Goes Across
Suture Lines

- Boggy edematous swelling of the fetal scalp.

- Disappears without treatment.

- No pathological significance.

CJMILLER

UMBILICAL CORD VESSELS

1 + 2 = 3
Vein   Arteries   Vessels

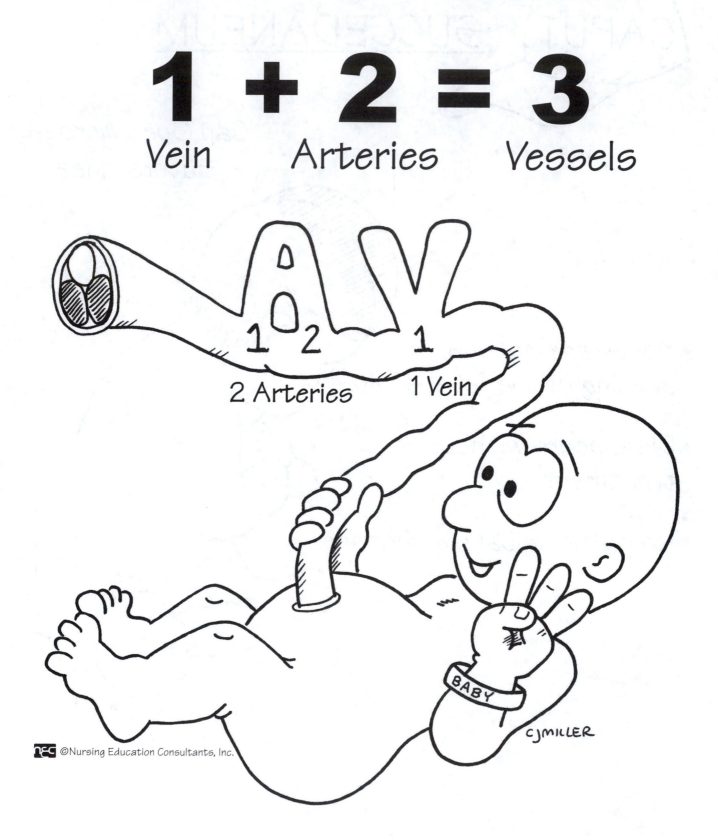

2 Arteries   1 Vein

©Nursing Education Consultants, Inc.

CJ MILLER

Maternity and Newborn
NursingEd.com

© 2012 Nursing Education
Consultants, Inc.

INDEX

© 2012 Nursing Education
Consultants, Inc.

Notes

Notes

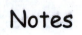

Notes

Notes